CANCER'S GIFT

by Donna L. Breen
edited by Michael Sion

Rock Wren Publishing
Reno, NV

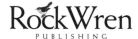

RockWren
PUBLISHING
P.O. Box 70326 - Reno, NV 89570-0326
(775) 829-4489 or toll-free (877) 481-8248
Fax: (775) 829-4459
rockwren@gbis.com

Copies of this book may be ordered from the publisher by sending $12.95
plus $4.75 for shipping and handling, or you may fax credit card information.

Publisher's Publication Data
Breen, Donna L. 1960 -
Cancer's Gift written by Donna L. Breen, 1st ed.,
with a foreword by Mark J. Mogul, M.D.

Summary: A family's journey through the world of cancer and
special relationships formed with other families and caregivers.

ISBN 0-9702238-0-3

1. Non-Fiction - Family & Relationships 2. Medical 3. Self-Help

Library of Congress Card Number: 00-191263

Cover and book design by Marnie Mattice

Printed in the United States of America

First Edition   10 9 8 7 6 5 4 3 2

Dedicated
to

Cassie, on her brand-new pink bike,
who continues to bring music to my life
at the most amazing times.

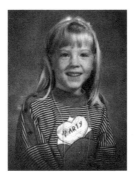

And to

Kendra, who will always soar like an eagle.

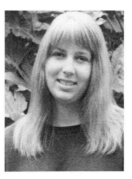

Thank you for teaching me the
meaning of courage and grace.

Illustrations with captions drawn by Anna Breen during Kyle's illness

Cover and chapter lettering contributed by Haley Breen

ACKNOWLEDGMENTS

Dr. Mark Mogul is the epitome of compassion and could be used as a model for all doctors hoping to reach out to their patients with love and understanding. Our entire family thanks God for Mark and his wonderful giving wife, Dr. Robin Mogul, and their beautiful son, Christopher.

My deepest love and gratitude to my entire family and our dear friends, who all rallied around us for the duration of Kyle's illness, regardless of what inconvenience it created for them and their families. Many people loved and cared for Anna while I was gone and Richmond was at work—often it was "Papa" and Leigh Miller and Deborah Smith. With special thanks to my sister, Dawn McMillin, who was there the first day Kyle and I stayed overnight in the hospital. Robin Shannon flew in to "baby-sit" me during an especially difficult time. And to my mom, Nola Jones, who flew in numerous times for six weeks at a time, putting her life in Dallas completely on hold so she could help care for Anna and our family.

Michael Sion, my editor extraordinaire, was brave and talented enough to take on this project. He is a pleasure to work with and his patience with my exuberance was greatly appreciated.

Marnie Mattice is insightful, incredibly generous and superbly talented in graphic design.

Kim and Jim Stone opened their home and hearts to us at a very trying time—A very brave move on their part. They were a godsend and helped us more than they'll ever know.

Dean Miller and Bill Highland graciously gave of their time and talent in the early stages of a very rough manuscript.

Bob, Joyce, Nicole and Tyson Lupro were bright lights on some of my darkest days. May we vacation together in tropical climates for the rest of our lives.

Many thanks to Sharon and David Green for their friendship and sharing their wonderful daughter, Kendra.

Grace Chamberlin Kelley, an incredible teacher, taught me to keep a journal. Its value during Kyle's illness was immeasurable. Often it was my only "friend" and allowed me to write things down that I would never have said out loud. It helped keep me sane.

Love and thanks to all the nurses and doctors for the compassion and courage it must take for them to care for patients on those really difficult days.

We are thankful for the incredible families we met at Children's Hospital at Stanford, and their friendship. And to the families we haven't met—embrace your new world. You will find friendship and good things in the most unlikely places.

Anna, Kyle and Haley's patience, love and support made this project possible. They are the best kids in the entire world.

My dear, sweet husband, Richmond, always encouraged me to take this project one step further. You, sweetheart, are without peer.

FOREWORD

On Aug. 15, 1997, I received a surprise telephone call. The call was from a 7-year-old boy who asked if I knew what was special about that day. When I replied I did not, he informed me that it marked his sixth year in remission from cancer. I proceeded to cry like a baby, and in a few moments my wife, who was next to me, was bawling, too, along with the boy's mother on the other end of the line.

The mother was Donna Breen; her son, Kyle. I was a month into a three-year pediatric oncology (childhood cancer) fellowship at Stanford Medical Center when I first encountered these two extraordinary people, seven years before. To say I am honored by the role I had to play in Kyle's well-being is an understatement. I am lucky to have been and to still be a part of this special family's lives.

I had started off my fellowship at Stanford totally naive. I had finished medical school at State University of New York, Syracuse, where I had decided during my junior year, during rotations at University Hospital in Syracuse, to specialize in pediatric oncology—treating children with cancer. I was drawn heart and soul to this field, with its intense personal approach to patients and their families, its emphasis on the human side of medicine. One physician in particular made a great impact on me. I saw him sit down with the shaken parents of a child who had just been diagnosed with a life-threatening illness. He carefully explained the child's condition, "No, your son is not dying tonight and, yes, there is something we can do about this." I realized, from how the parents hung on his every word, what an incredibly important role oncologists play.

When I picked up Kyle's case a month into my fellowship at Stanford, I fancied myself as an Albert Schweitzer, able to cure everyone I touched. This, of course, is not reality in the field of medicine, and particularly in a cancer ward. I had much to learn. Donna was among the first people to really impress upon me what it means to have a child with cancer. She and her husband, Richmond, are educated, articulate people who love their children unconditionally. Both are very earthy people, practitioners of healthy lifestyles and naturally repelled by chemotherapy, which they regarded as poison. Yet, once convinced their infant son could only fight his cancer by receiving chemotherapy and radiation therapy, they went along with the program.

The cancer Kyle had, was called neuroblastoma. This disease has about a 90 percent cure rate when it presents in infancy. As expected, Kyle's tumor responded very well to therapy, and it was a shock when the tumor relapsed. Donna has explained the process of fighting cancer from a layperson's perspective. She not only records her experiences—how Kyle's treatment impacted her—with precision, but accurately explains the medical care in minute detail. Reading her manuscript, I was deeply impressed by how much she understood. She also relates the key lessons about life that dealing with cancer impart.

During my training, I came to value what great teachers young patients themselves are, with their absolute honesty and their zest for life in the face of grim circumstances. I found that even children as young as 4 or 5 realize the importance of the therapy they undergo, and will endure whatever it takes to get them better. If you were to tell them to stand on their heads four hours a day, they would do it. They mature so quickly. And many are worried not for their own welfare but how their disease impacts their parents. Gosh, if I don't make it, how can I make this easier on my parents?

I remember one girl, Heather—a roommate of another young woman, Kendra, whom Donna writes about in this book. Heather was undergoing experimental therapy for a bone-marrow transplant. She was receiving chemotherapy with Mitoxantrone, a bright-blue substance which she called, "Mito-Tidy Bowl." She hoped it would get her into remission. The first cell that popped up in her blood smear was a leukemia cell. It was clear at that point there was nothing else we could do. After I broke the news to her family, I went to have a conversation with her alone. She said, "Mark, how old are you?" I said 28. She said, "Twenty-eight. I'm never going to get there. I want to play bingo when I'm 80." She wanted to live and do things, to have her first boyfriend—all those milestones.

It was another of the constant reminders about how precious life is, and how much it means for these kids to get out of the hospital and back home to be with their family and friends. Fortunately, we cure more kids than we don't. Irrespective of the number of children we treat, it is horrible for us when a child dies. What keeps us going, however, is that at least half of all children with cancer are cured, and even in the worst cases, we can make a positive difference for a patient and his or her family. How do you put into words what it's like to have children come back year after year for checkups after they had been virtually on death's door, and now they're healthy with their whole lives ahead of them? How can you underestimate the importance of that?

This explains the emotional reaction I and my wife had to Kyle's phone call that summer day.

Donna's book is important for several kinds of readers. Foremost, it will help those with children entering a cancer ward to understand that they're not alone in feeling overwhelmed, even as they are shocked, frightened and unprepared for what lies ahead, and deluged with information they can't begin to immediately absorb. This book will assure them that in time, they'll be amazed how much they'll comprehend about their child's medical care—just as Donna learned it's no big deal to handle a catheter.

This book also is a valuable document for health-care professionals to better understand their field and the perspectives of patients and their families. And finally, this is an important book for people in general, for the reader cannot help but feel like a part of Donna's family by sharing her experience.

The lessons contained within these pages are essential; namely, the importance of the love of family and of friends, and the faith that we all have the opportunity to make the most of our lives—including to be there for our fellow humans through both the good and bad.

These are life's great lessons.

MARK J. MOGUL, M.D.

CONTENTS

CHAPTER 1

AT THE BEGINNING

It was August 1990 when our lives took a dramatic turn. We were in the bloom of familyhood. My husband, Richmond—33, athletic and tanned—was busy running his landscaping business. I was 30, and enjoying the luxury of staying home with our children after seven years in the roofing industry. Anna was a beautiful, energetic 2-year-old with blond curls like her father. Kyle, born in May, was a chubby, good-natured baby.

One Saturday, on our way home down the mountain to Reno from an outing at Lake Tahoe, Anna began throwing up. At home that evening she developed a fever. But the illness passed almost as quickly as it came, and she was back to normal in a few days.

The next Saturday, Kyle seemed like he had the flu. No big surprise. Anna loved to kiss her little brother, so we had expected him to get sick. Then, Sunday afternoon, he stopped urinating. This was disturbing. I tried to reach our pediatrician, Dr. Patrick Colletti. His telephone answering exchange relayed my message to another doctor on call, who suspected dehydration and recommended fluids. So I tried nursing Kyle every hour or two through the night, but he wasn't very interested in eating. In the morning, his diaper was still dry.

Our concern now growing, we took him to Dr. Colletti. He immediately said Kyle would have to go into the hospital for an "IV and hydration." Without specifying reasons, the pediatrician made it clear that Kyle required care that an office visit could not provide. I remember thinking how terrible a discomfort an intravenous tube would be for this poor little baby. The flu, diarrhea and vomiting were bad enough. Kyle was less than 3 months old.

On Tuesday, Kyle was admitted to Saint Mary's Regional Medical Center, in Reno. Dr. Colletti showed up promptly and took Kyle to the treatment room where IV starts are performed, and got a line started in a vein in our baby's head. I was stunned. I couldn't believe our infant son was in the hospital. He lay in the steel crib with a mesh cap covering the IV tube taped to his head. He looked so tiny and vulnerable I felt like grabbing him and running away—anywhere.

Dr. Colletti also catheterized Kyle to check for fluid in his bladder. It was so full we were probably lucky it hadn't popped. They took out 300 cubic centimeters (cc) of urine. For comparison: the average adult first feels the urge to urinate at 250 cc, which becomes more of a need at 300 cc.

After running a few more tests, Dr. Colletti sent us to a urologist, Dr. Bruce Wallace. He was about Dr. Colletti's age, in his early 40s, with dark hair. He was easy to talk to and Richmond and I felt comfortable asking questions. My first questions were when Kyle could come home, and what might be wrong with him. After examining Kyle, Dr. Wallace suggested a non-invasive surgery to see if there was a blockage preventing urination. A non-invasive surgery entails very little, if any, cutting by the surgeon. This was what we all hoped for: a "quick fix."

On Thursday, Dr. Wallace performed the exploratory operation. He found no conclusive findings, and in a second surgery gave Kyle a "supra pubic tube." This is a tube inserted through the abdominal wall to empty the urine from the bladder. The tube seemed to be made of rubber or latex and was about 1/4-inch wide and 2 feet long with a bag at the end to catch urine. Both surgeries were completed that morning in about an hour, though it seemed much longer to us. Upon returning to his room, Kyle seemed spent, though not upset or in pain.

At this point I felt overwhelmed. Staring at our infant in a hospital bed with tubes coming out of him left me fearful and stunned. Being unfamiliar with the tubes, I was afraid to pick up my baby. Feelings of inadequacy rushed over me with the realization that my abilities to heal my son were meager. Dr. Wallace came to speak to me while I stood by Kyle's bed.

"You can take Kyle home in the morning," he said. "We'll watch him for a week to 10 days to see if he starts urinating on his own. Although this is a long shot."

"I can't take my baby home," I replied, "until you take this tube out!"

Dr. Wallace kindly reassured me. He said keeping Kyle in the hospital for two weeks was not practical. I remember thinking he was crazy, that he must have overestimated me. How could I possibly take care of that tube sticking out of Kyle's belly? But Dr. Wallace explained it to me. A few times a day the tube needed to be swabbed clean, and ointment applied to the opening. Simple enough, in retrospect.

Richmond and I were confident Kyle's ailment was merely a blip on our family screen. This trouble would just "go away," we told each other. Dr. Wallace and Dr. Colletti suggested an MRI (Magnetic Resonance Image) while we waited. An MRI bounces magnetic waves off the body, allowing different tissue masses to be identified. A woman I saw at Idelwild pool regularly with her two small children, said her husband, a radiologist, read MRIs, and wanted more experience. He offered to read it, free of charge. We thought that was really nice: and the bills were already snowballing, even though we had great insurance. Principal Mutual had been easy to work with and though we had already spent a few thousand dollars of our own money, Principal had kept up its end of the insurance agreement. But then again, was there really a need for this? Richmond and I canceled the MRI.

Dr. Colletti and Dr. Wallace urged us to reschedule the examination. Without denial clouding their judgment, they could see there was an unidentified problem that needed to be rectified. More information was needed. We acquiesced.

We let our acquaintance read it. Anyone standing on the outside would have been shaking his head over our resistance and our choice of letting someone with so little experience read our son's test. But remember: We had no experience. The tests results read: "Nothing abnormal."

The next few days, Richmond's and my thoughts and conversations went back and forth. *Our child was fine... Wasn't he?*

Gee what's that tube for? No problem. He just can't urinate. Oh, he's fine, it's just a virus. He'll be fine in a couple of days.

Hello! Wow! Denial can get thick. Our baby had a tube coming out of his abdomen, no ability to urinate on his own, yet we were working hard to convince ourselves nothing was wrong!

A few days later we called Dr. Wallace back. He, in no uncertain terms, recommended we admit Kyle into a teaching hospital for further tests, because they are on the cutting edge of research. From his tone, I think he was ready to drive us there himself.

We believed in our hearts that Kyle was OK. Did we really need to go to a research hospital? Dr. Colletti and Dr. Wallace were steadfast. "Go! Go to a teaching hospital and get Kyle checked out," Dr. Colletti said.

Not too long after that I wrote them both notes, thanking them for being such great doctors. They both had the courage to say, "I don't know, you need to find someone that does." That's the kind of doctors we wanted, ones confident and competent enough to know when to pass the ball. We were so grateful.

During that time, Richmond's father, Fran, an outdoorsman in his seventies and a Stanford University law graduate, had been encouraging us to take Kyle for a second opinion. "Take him down to Stanford!" he said. "They've got a great children's hospital and an incredible research facility."

He was right.

Believing Kyle didn't have any real problems, I told Richmond, "Stanford's only five hours away. Kyle and I will go and you can keep working. I'll only be a few days." My stepmother, Leigh, was going to watch Anna while I was gone. I knew I could handle a few tests. No problem. I gathered the records of the tests already performed and drove down to Palo Alto, Calif., the next day, Sept. 12. It was a lovely drive, crossing Donner Summit, the Sacramento Valley and the Bay Bridge into San Francisco.

WHILE DRIVING, I THOUGHT about when Richmond and I had met in Reno, four years before.

We were in our twenties, full of life, excitement and great hopes for the future.

Introduced over coffee one morning by Bonnie Learey, a mutual friend, I listened to Richmond talk and was thunderstruck by his presence. My mind was aflutter. On our way out of the restaurant, he put his arm around my shoulder and hugged me. As he left, I whispered to Bonnie, "Oh my God, I have to see him again." He had already suggested we come see the raised stone flower beds he was doing for the Roberts, who were both family friends and clients. So later that day we swung by the job site, "to see the work he was doing." I felt like a schoolgirl when he asked me out to dinner later that week.

After dating plenty of guys, Mr. Right had continued to elude me. But from our first meeting it was clear Richmond was special.

We went to dinner at Mama's Cantina and had a wonderful time. We talked about our interests, likes and dislikes and our jobs. I couldn't believe what I was hearing. It was as if he were made for me. In my mind I was checking off the "requirements for the man I marry." I couldn't check them off quickly enough. Marriage and kids were at the top of the list. So was staying at home with the kids or perhaps working part-time. Gardening and cooking food that we had grown were also common interests. A farm wasn't on my list, but raising some animals for food—his intention—sounded intriguing. Check, check, check, and check again. He was perfect!

At the time, roofing was my occupation. Returning to college was also a consideration, though I was enjoying my work. After being an office receptionist for the roofing company and seeing the difference in paychecks, I decided at 22 to give roofing a try. After four years of apprenticeship, I received my journeyman's card from the largest roofing union in the country. I worked on industrial buildings and high-rises doing hot tar, rubber and vinyl flat roofs for Roofers Union Local 11. I worked hard and learned everything I could about the trade, wanting to be one of the best in the business. Being the only woman in an 1,800-member union was challenging. It took six months before some of the men would even let me sit with them for a coffee break. The Chicago roofers are not a mellow bunch. They are a rough group, and many have "done time" behind bars. On top of that, the weather in the Windy City could be brutal with hot, muggy summers and winters that are cold, windy and damp. Ninety-five percent of the men acted pretty decently toward me after they realized I could do my job. Being able to carry 100 pounds of materials, along with what tools I had around my waist, up a ladder often wasn't enough. With a group of men that rough you needed an attitude. My motto was, "Get tough or die."

At 5-foot-2, 110 pounds I wasn't a knockout, but hadn't been hit with "the ugly stick" either. Some men found the combination of looks and skill intimidating. My future spouse would have to be confident and flexible.

And there I was now, sitting across the restaurant table from the potentially perfect husband. I couldn't believe it. It was only our first date, but being a very direct person, I cut to the chase.

"If you don't want to get married and have kids within a year," I said, "I don't even want to date you."

Mind you, it was like Richmond was trapped in a booth and I'd shot him with a stun gun. His face dropped a bit, his lips parted slightly and a blank expression crossed his face for a few moments. Upon recovery he didn't even break into the 100-yard dash. He just sat there and muttered, "Well ... if we get along."

Dating people that weren't marriage material was tiring. Falling in love with someone whose goals weren't the same was a trap that was avoidable with open communication. I wasn't serious about my timetable but simply wanted him to know I was serious about my future.

We continued to date, vacation together, and spend a lot of our day-to-day lives together. We fell madly in love and couldn't imagine being apart. Within a few months we announced to our families that we would be married in the fall of 1987.

AFTER FIVE HOURS OF driving and daydreaming, I pulled into the tree-lined campus of Stanford University. Flower beds paved the way toward the medical center, where beautiful rolling hills and an upscale shopping center lay on the immediate outskirts. At the medical center, we were first seen by a urologist, then sent across the street to Children's Hospital at Stanford for a sonogram. A friendly young woman named Michelle was the technologist. After she rubbed some ultrasound gel on Kyle's abdomen, she ran the scanner over his pelvic region. The gel acts as a conductor for the scanner to read noise frequencies that outline internal organs and tissues in the body, producing a picture similar to an X-ray. The picture is visible for a radiologist to read almost immediately. I could tell Michelle was sharp and had lots of experience. She completed her task and wiped the gel off Kyle's belly, all the while making polite conversation.

"So, what do you see?" I asked as I munched a turkey sandwich.

"Oh, I don't know," she replied. "I'm just a tech."

I believed she could read the results on the screen in front of her, but I knew it was not her job to deliver this information.

The doctor came in a few minutes later as I was finishing my sandwich. He was young, tall and slender with short auburn hair and a compassionate expression. His gaze met mine as he sat down across from me and started to speak.

"There is a mass," he said quietly.

"A mass?!" I asked. "What's a mass? A mass of what?"

"It's a tumor in his pelvis," he continued. "It's about the size of a baseball."

Oh my God! A tumor! No matter how you say it, "a tumor" just doesn't sound good.

It occurred to me that I had better start writing some of this down, since things were getting a little complicated. I had brought stationery with me, intending to write a letter to my grandma or grandpa. Nice thought.

After a full day of tests and tromping through the halls of the Stanford Medical Center and Children's Hospital, Kyle and I were beat. We checked into the Hyatt. I ordered an entrée and glass of wine from room service and tried to think of how to break the news to Richmond.

Sitting on the bed, I made an effort to absorb what I had been told that day. It was unbelievable that Kyle had a tumor. Stunned, overcome with dread, I found myself not wanting to call Richmond. How could I tell him that his son had a tumor? There just wasn't any easy way to do it. I finally dialed, after Kyle was settled in, around 5 p.m.

"Hello," he said, and immediately asked, "how did the tests go today?"

"I don't know quite how to say this ... Kyle has a tumor."

The silence from his end was overwhelming. Finally, he began firing questions. "Are you sure? What did they say? What kind of tumor is it? Is it malignant?"

"They don't know what it is," I answered. "They want to do more tests tomorrow. Kyle is going to have a CAT scan as soon as they can fit us in. We'll go back first thing in the morning."

Richmond paused. Almost whispering, he asked, "Are you all right?"

"I'm O.K. ..." I reassured him. "Everyone's been very nice. We'll be home tomorrow after they finish the tests. After all ... it could be benign. It's got to be benign."

Our relatives hoped for the same. Whether it was Richmond or myself who called them that night remains a vague memory. We both agreed that the Hyatt was money well spent. Richmond felt terrible that I was down there by myself. But never for a moment did I feel deserted, or upset with my husband. My being a strong person was a definite plus, and I reassured him that I was fine. After all, we would be home the next day. Kyle was scheduled for an IV and CAT scan in the morning. After that we would come home. It would be a long day but I could certainly handle it by myself.

The next morning I waited nervously in a small waiting room at Stanford University Hospital, wishing the tests results were in, and wanting to be at home where I felt safe and protected. All of the uncertainty was frightening and shook me to my core.

THAT NEXT MORNING AT the hospital, I made what was to be the first entry in a journal I would keep for the duration of the crisis. The stationery I wrote on had been intended for much lighter subject matter.

> 9/13/90 9:00 a.m.
> *We sit and wait for IV's and dye for Kyle's CAT scan. We don't know when they'll take us, but they are squeezing us in, and we are thankful for that. We listened to excellent music on the way to the hospital, rockin' out. We can enjoy the morning, we have the whole day to fall apart.*
>
> *We didn't expect a tumor. We were sure this was a fluke. Don't throw rocks at my glass house, Please. Now we are sure it's benign. It better be.*
>
> *I pray so much. How many prayers do you suppose are said as people turn into the entrance at the Children's Hospital? God must have a direct line—I hope so.*

We were sent to Day Hospital to wait for tests. Day Hospital is an outpatient clinic in Children's Hospital for kids who need an IV of medication or a blood transfusion. There were a number of rooms off the main area, each with televisions, beds and windows. Many of the rooms had children in them, each with his or her own IV pole holding some kind of medicine, or pint bags of blood.

Holding Kyle, I overheard a conversation about Cheetos making some boy feel better. It seemed as this boy's IV dripped, he started throwing up. He casually took the barf holder and said, "Oh well, there go the Cheetos." Sitting there, realizing these kids were getting chemotherapy, left me awestruck and unable to imagine why we were waiting in there. I must of had that, "I have no idea my kid is *really* sick" look on my face. I was amazed by the conversations around me. Moms were discussing broccoli and laundry. Didn't they know where they were? It was unbelievable! Life was going on for them.

Journal entries from that longest day of my motherhood sum up the stormy waves of thoughts crashing through my mind:

> **9/13/90   11:00 a.m.**
> *How many days in a row with cramps from stress. I can't leave his side. There are lots of children crying. I am crying. This is a hard place to be. I want to go home. I love you Richmond. I love you Anna. I need you and thank God I have you.*

> **9/13/90   Midnight**
> *It is very late. Everyone we know and love is stunned. I am shocked. This has been a lot of stress on Kyle's body. The exams don't seem to quit. A poke here a prod there. We of older ages would be making a lot of complaining noises.*
>
> *Maybe tomorrow we will have more information, Richmond (RHB) thinks Mom should fly in. I think he's right. Tomorrow is new day and we will survive.*

The next morning, as I sat on a blue-cushioned chair in the waiting room for CAT scans, I watched a physician approach. He appeared to be in his mid 40s, balding, with glasses and a placid demeanor. He sat down and looked at me with a kind expression.

"I'm Dr. Gary Hartman," he said. "Kyle's CAT scan is finished. I do quite a few of these and I'm 90 percent sure it's a tumor called neuroblastoma."

"Are we talking about the 'C' word here?"

"I'm afraid so," he answered.

Devastated, I mulled over the information. My first question was, "What is the prognosis?"

In a calm voice, he said, "We have very good success with neuroblastoma."

The male and female nurse wore concerned expressions as they stood with hands folded casually together as I was told Kyle had cancer. Had they sent an extra nurse along just to sedate me? That would have been totally unnecessary. Instantaneous shock had set in, leaving me quite calm. The nurses suggested my husband drive down immediately. I told them to forget it. Navigating the Bay Area's traffic requires all one's faculties. The last thing I needed was my husband getting killed in a wreck because he was so upset. Kyle and I got in our car and returned to the Hyatt.

As soon as I got him situated in the center of the king-size bed, I called room service.

"I want two glasses of chardonnay sent up right away," I said. "I just found out my baby has cancer and I need a sedative."

Telling this to a total stranger was odd; hearing it come out of my mouth and knowing it was the truth was almost like an out-of-body experience.

I hung up and stood there dazed, wondering how in the world I would be able to pass on the news. I wandered around the room, trying to get my thoughts together before calling Richmond. As I paced the floor, it occurred to me that I hadn't even given room service my number. I dialed again. The man who answered said, "Oh, thank God you called back, we've been frantically trying to figure out what room you called from. We'll be right up."

Kyle had an IV in his leg. It could be reused if I "locked it" with heparin, an anti-clogging medicine. The only requirement was to swab off the tube with an alcohol wipe and inject a needle with heparin in it. The needle went not in his skin but the tube. Being very inexperienced, and the baby being very squirmy, I felt unable to accomplish this task alone. I considered my available resources. The room service guy showed up and I told him—in a firm command that left him no option to decline—"Hold the baby's leg, I have to give him this injection." The dark-haired young man in his early 20s was pretty flustered but did as he was told. With the heparin lock complete, I signed for room service and said, "Thank you."

Calling Richmond that evening was the hardest thing I had ever done. Cancer is associated with death. I told him in a soft, steady voice that the doctor had said, in these exact words, "There are lots of success stories." We tried to keep that thought in the forefront, but fear was pushing hard at our optimism. We talked at length and decided who would call whom to inform our family. Richmond's dad, Fran, was at our house, along with my step-mom, Leigh, who had watched Anna that day, and my dad, Dick Miller. Dad is thin, of medium height, with graying hair. I hoped his heart would hold up under the news. Richmond and I hung up; he was faced with the job of breaking the news to Fran, Dad, Leigh and little Anna.

It was after this conversation that our long-distance phone bill truly went sky-high. Richmond and I were both on long-distance and local calls for six hours that night. There wasn't a good or quick way to tell friends and family that our baby had cancer. Yet I didn't cry once. I had to be strong, to convey hope and courage.

I needed to sleep. It came easy.

> **9/14/90 6:30 a.m.**
> *We (Kyle and I) woke up, and find the day has not begun as we expected. We expect to wake up from this nightmare but haven't.*

SINCE THE NIGHTMARE WAS still running, we gathered our-selves, got some breakfast in the restaurant and drove off toward the hospital. I stared stone-faced through the windshield. Some sappy love song came on the radio—and that's when the dam burst. Suddenly, my body felt as if it weren't my own. I came unglued. Convulsing with sobs, moaning and crying out loud, I pulled over and stopped the car.

I wept and cried out, "Oh my God. No! Not my baby!"

After several minutes I gathered myself, and pulled back into morning traffic. Moments later the wave of anguish came crashing in again. Kyle, his child safety seat set facing the car's interior in the passenger side of our Toyota pickup, watched me the entire time, seemingly unaffected.

Pulling into Children's Hospital, I said a prayer at the entrance and sat in the parking lot getting myself together. It took about 15 minutes of deep breathing. Looking into the rearview mirror, deep rings and red, swollen eyes stared back at me with a strange, distant look: almost those of another person.

I knew it was time to center myself.

I realized this was the first morning in some time I had woken without stomach cramps from stress. I considered that sometimes the not knowing is worse than the knowing. It had been almost a month since Kyle first became ill. Finally, at least, we were getting some answers.

CHAPTER 2

A WHOLE NEW WORLD

Walking into Children's Hospital the morning after the crushing news, not knowing what treatment was planned for Kyle, felt like entering a foreign country. I was totally apprehensive and disoriented. Luckily, Kyle was still happy as could be.

He was an easy baby who bounced back quickly from physical discomforts and continued to be cheerful and full of smiles. I carried him to the desk at Clinic D and told Marcia, the receptionist, who we were. She was a heavyset woman with dark curly hair and a serious, but kind, voice. Watching her, it was clear to me that she was an integral part of the nerve center at the oncology clinic. In her businesslike fashion she said she knew who we were and was expecting us. Boy, that was it—they knew us already. We were now part of this strange world.

The dam burst, again, and out came the tears.

Marcia asked me to sit down. She said the wait wouldn't be too long. I found ourselves in a room full of people who had already been through this. I sobbed and rocked Kyle. A boy about 12 said to a companion, "I remember when my parents found out I had cancer. They were really bummed." I couldn't believe what I was hearing! *They were really bummed*. Here was a kid on chemo, already spending his days in a cancer ward, talking as if he had a broken arm. That was the first moment that I thought, "If he can go through this with that attitude, maybe I can help Kyle through."

Kyle and I were sent to an examining room to wait for his doctor. As I leafed through a children's book I started laughing my head off, as if I'd gone half-crazy. Yet the laughter felt like a soothing tonic. It was then that I realized humor is a terrific coping mechanism.

In walked Dr. Mark Mogul with his dark wavy hair, medium build, and great smile. At 30, he possessed a youthful enthusiasm. Under his name-tag it read, "Fellow." Not knowing that was a reference to seniority in the medical world, all I could think was, Would anyone really think he was a girl?

"Hi, my name is Mark Mogul," he said. "I'll be Kyle's doctor when you come in here."

Here was a man whose services we would need desperately, and I replied, "Oh, no. Don't tell me I'm going to have to look at your face every time we come in."

"Most parents feel that way," he said, not missing a beat. "But they get over it."

So this was it. We officially had an oncologist, and I'd already insulted him. Thank God he came with a great sense of humor. If he was half as nice as he seemed to be, we were going to be working with the cream of the crop. His manner was very patient and I felt he would have stayed all day answering my numerous questions if I'd needed him to.

So far, everyone we had dealt with had treated us with kindness and respect. I felt good about the care Kyle was getting. Children's Hospital even had a transportation staff on call, if you had to get to a building that was distant or difficult to find in the complex. Everyone we met in transport was wonderful. They were always cheerful and would talk to Kyle and try to make him smile.

After a full day of testing, Kyle and I hopped in our truck and drove home. It was 5 p.m., and the last time I was to drive home that late. A five-hour drive over a serious mountain pass was too much when the day had been so taxing. But the drive proved uneventful and we were happy and relieved to pull in at home.

> **9/15 Saturday night—Dawn flies in**
> *Thank God for family. You know it's bad when a sister who never takes time away from her family flies out to help. I'm so glad she's here.*

Dawn is my older sister but we could almost pass for twins. After flying in from Chicago, she was going back to Children's with me so Richmond could keep working. We all had jobs now.

His was to keep the business going so we could pay our bills. No one waved the magic wand to make the bills go away. Anna spent a lot of time with my dad and Leigh. My sister-in-law, Deborah Smith, and her husband, Mike, also lived in Reno and took Anna frequently. The formative years are so important, and I worried I wasn't spending enough time with her. She was doing well so far and getting lots of attention. I was the hospital person. It was a good thing as I was simply better at it. I have teased Richmond, calling him "nature boy." He is a man who never takes an aspirin unless he is wrecked, and now our son was going to the land of chemical therapy. We only had the weekend to regroup, but it was something. Two "normal" days as an intact family unit, before Kyle would have to return to Stanford for a tissue biopsy—and the beginning of chemo.

DAWN AND I TOOK our time driving to Stanford on Monday. Dawn was in charge of amusing Kyle on the way. We had a little plastic bath book that she claimed emitted "sleeping gas," because every time she showed it to him he fell asleep. It made us laugh. We stopped off in San Francisco and relaxed over a nice lunch with some wine in a wonderful restaurant overlooking the Bay.

As we drove on to Stanford, Dawn and I talked about my career in roofing and my marriage. I had been offered a job by a roofing manufacturer based in Chicago. The company managers had already met me during my union years and were interested in having me cover the western states as a technical representative. The money was good and the job was a lot cleaner than installing roofs. I was the only woman in their company who wasn't in a clerical position. The attire was business suits and the language wasn't nearly as colorful as it was on the roof, but it was still a male-dominated field and required mental toughness. And I enjoyed my new job, often flying three days a week to visit sites and troubleshoot and consult. As before, 95 percent of the men were very nice and treated me with respect, but the remaining 5 percent could really be buggers.

Richmond and I were married in September as planned, and had a fantastic ceremony and reception. We have always enjoyed life to the fullest and rather than waiting, tried right away to have children. We were successful. I became pregnant in a very short time. We had a problem-free pregnancy and delivery. Anna Adair Breen was born in May 18, 1988. Her middle name was after Robin Adair Shannon, my best friend since we were 7. Robin was now a nurse, a beautiful redhead with a casual, confident manner. Adair was Robin's maiden name.

Along with Anna came all the beauty of parenthood. We were amazed, thrilled and tired. I had three months off work, and intended to go back three days a week. Robin visited two weeks before I was to return to the job. She brought her 6-month-old baby, Ryan. I cried so much just thinking about going back to work that when Richmond got home from his deer hunt, he said, "Don't go back. We'll do fine." When I called the roofing company to resign I got a pleasant surprise. The company offered me eight hours a week, spread out if I needed it. It was an offer I couldn't pass up. The next year-and-a-half I helped my employers build a new manufacturing plant in Fernley, a community neighboring Reno. As the only local rep, I oversaw construction, sending reports and photos back to Chicago.

I hung up my roofing hatchet and briefcase during the last trimester of my pregnancy with Kyle. It had been eight years in a field that had challenged me physically and mentally. Three years were spent as a tech, and though I don't care to install roofing again, I wouldn't change a bit of that strenuous experience, either. Looking back, I realized it was good training for the more difficult challenges that lay ahead. It got me used to coping with stress for long periods.

Dawn, Kyle and I arrived at Children's Hospital and checked in. We were sent down to the Auxiliary ward/Cancer ward, Room 402. There were four beds with a child in each, and parents sitting near three of the four. I began unpacking, trying not to stare at the other children. The unpacking didn't take long, and we had nothing to do but sit.

The boy in the bed across was about 11. He was missing an arm and an eye, and part of his cheek bone. He didn't say a word. In the bed kitty-corner from me was a 6-year-old girl who never moved a muscle. Her name was Cassie Lupro. Cassie had a younger sister, Nicole, with dark hair and a sparkling personality. Her older brother, Tyson, was tall and thin with a warm smile. Bob and Joyce were her parents. They were in their late 30s, casual and calm, and appeared to know the ropes in this macabre setting.

Seasoned veterans, they flew in from Juneau, Alaska. The distance they traveled put my drive into perspective right away.

The other bed had a 4-year-old girl in it. She was newly diagnosed and screamed if anyone even walked by the door. She was terrified of "pokes"—shots.

Dawn and I were mortified by this setting. I couldn't see how I could handle it for days or weeks at a stretch. The nurse came in and let me know about the Teddy Bear Phone—a phone mounted in the middle of a big, tan, stuffed bear attached to the wall halfway down a corridor. The Teddy Bear Phone was free, anywhere, anytime, courtesy of a major long distance carrier. (Needless to say, it came to save us hundreds of dollars. A godsend!)

But I was too shaken to appreciate the Teddy Bear Phone at that moment. I walked down the hall full of gloom. How could I possibly live through this hell? I called Richmond and just started crying. "I can't stay here. I can't do this."

I knew in my heart there wasn't a choice, but I was overpowered by fear. Richmond, not really knowing what to say, reassured me as much as possible. And what, indeed, could he say?

After hanging up, I walked back to our room, stopping along the way to ask the nurse when we could get a private room. She said that a room with two beds would perhaps open up, but usually the private rooms were full. What she didn't say was that the kids in private rooms were so sick it wouldn't be mentally healthy for anyone else to room with them. They were dying. As I later learned, those rooms were reserved; and we certainly didn't want a reservation.

Back at our room, I couldn't stop crying.

"You don't have to stay," Dawn said. "You could come back to the hotel with me. Kyle's little. He won't know you're gone."

This was unbelievable coming from Dawn. She never left her girls for anything. I thought about it and realized that if I didn't stay at the hospital that night, I never would. I would just have to be tough in this chamber of cancer.

As we were sitting bedside, in walked Kendra Green. Kendra was 15, a very pretty brunette, athletic, and with a wonderful personality. She had a tumor called rhabdomyosarcoma. Kendra's mom, Sharon, was standing behind her holding the IV pole and looking like she'd been run over by a semi. Kendra gave us her best Valley Girl description of chemo:

"Chemo's not that bad. On my worst day I only threw up six times and had three dry heaves. No big deal."

I couldn't believe it! Here was a 15-year-old girl with an incredible attitude and gift to spread cheer and courage at just the right moment. I knew then, that we could do it. What an inspiration. She had just finished some chemo and was not impressed. She was going the mile and nothing was going to get her down.

A little later, Dawn left. I felt much better, and though I didn't sleep well that night, I was starting to feel a little less overcome with despair. Each of the four sections of the room had a curtain that pulled around on a track to provide some privacy. Standing behind that curtain changing into my jammies drove home to me the fact that the Children's cancer ward was our new "home." I was less than comfortable with our accommodations, but I knew my comfort was the least of our worries. Unfolding the rollaway cot, I made my bed with the clean sheets and blanket the nurse had given me out of the closet down the hall. I laid down to sleep next to a sink that dripped through the night. Ironic, I thought, as I understood dripping water is an old form of torture.

It was like having 10 people in my bedroom when I woke up. I had "bed hair." I was in my jammies and slippers and hadn't had a cup of coffee or brushed my teeth. Normally, I did all of these things before seeing anyone other than family. It was very awkward for me when a group of five or six residents came by about 7:30 a.m. for morning rounds. I knew I would rise, shower and dress a lot earlier in the future to minimize my personal discomfort with "everyone being in my bedroom." I got myself together and ran down to the cafeteria for a to-go plate. "Breakfast of champions," hospital food was not! However, scrambled eggs and fresh fruit are a pretty safe bet. Dinners of mystery meat and gravy were something I stayed away from.

My sister arrived and Kyle's day of tests began. The tissue biopsy was done by a surgeon. A large needle—about the size of fat spaghetti—was stuck through his rectum wall into the tumor, and tissue was extracted for a biopsy test. The pediatric surgical team was Dr. Gary Hartman and Dr. Steven Schocat. Dr. Schocat was in his 40s, with a pleasant but businesslike manner. Each physician had a fantastic reputation.

By that evening we had received results of Kyle's bone scan and bone marrow smear. They had come back clear. We were still waiting for a bone biopsy and a test in which they would send his urine to a lab in Oklahoma—though I could hardly believe that. I was grateful how soundly Kyle slept on morphine. It had dripped through his IV prior to the tissue biopsy to eliminate his pain. I had a different "tranquilizer": an exercise bike which sat in the hallway outside a room next to ours. Peddling for about 20 minutes helped alleviate some stress, and at the same time, seemed to humor the nurses at a nearby station.

We were at the beginning of a long frightening journey fraught with many unknowns. I chose to concentrate on the positive—they hadn't just shaken our hands and sent us home with no chance of survival. Kyle *had* a chance. That was all that mattered.

We met a number of people in the short time we had been there who were coping very well and maintained a great sense of humor. Again, a coping mechanism. One was a mother of a 3-year-old named Matthew. He had lost an eye due to cancer, but it didn't slow him down and with a hat on and no IV pole he would pass for any other 3-year-old. He definitely kept his mom hopping. He had a false eye that he had learned to pop out. One day they were at the local grocery store and she heard carts crashing and Matthew laughing. He had rolled his eye down the aisle and the shoppers were mortified. If that wasn't bad enough, she had to retrieve it from under a big potato chip rack.

"Oh excuse me…Manager…my son's eye is under your display, could you help me?" Kids are truly amazing!

I called Richmond and Anna every day from the Teddy Bear Phone. Though my attitude was much improved from the first night, he was still very concerned about how I was holding up during Kyle's care. Poor Richmond! Dawn, Kyle and I came pulling in that Wednesday evening and instead of fear, out poured stories punctuated with hysterical bouts of laughter. I'm sure he thought we had gone completely nuts. We'd tell a story and laugh uncontrollably. I'm surprised he didn't send for the straitjackets. Richmond has a good sense of humor, but he was just so flabbergasted and shocked at our behavior he didn't know what to say. He thought we'd driven right over the edge. Indeed—given our stress—it was probably a short drive. Our laughter was a result of the built-up anxiety.

My mom, Nola, had offered to fly in from Dallas the moment this whole nightmare started. Mom was a strong, compassionate yet realistic woman in her 60s. We were very close. But I didn't feel as if I needed the help yet. I had spent many years in a profession that taught me to be fiercely independent. I tried to never ask for help, but to accomplish my goals on my own. Yet I was beginning to flounder. Richmond and I were a great team, but the new game plan seemed to required some extra players.

One morning I called Mom from the Teddy Bear Phone. "I'm coming out Thursday," she offered.

I was so relieved to hear this. Then Dean, my brother, came in from Wyoming the same day. Dean is handsome, with light-brown wavy hair and a lean build. He is an outdoorsman, more independent than I, and has a tremendous heart. We gathered together and spent the next few days having some fun. Lake Tahoe was magnificent. We spent a day at a friend's house right on the water. It was a welcome reprieve, for the same Thursday my mother and brother arrived, Dr. Mogul had phoned. Kyle was officially diagnosed with neuroblastoma.

Our baby had a malignant tumor! The doctors had mentioned many options to us regarding the approach to Kyle's care. Surgery was suggested to remove as much of the baseball-sized tumor as possible. We agreed. Richmond and I would both be at Stanford while Mom and Dean stayed with Anna. It was reassuring to know that our daughter would be sleeping in her own bed and eating lunch in her own house. So far, her life had been severely disrupted. Anna was one of my biggest concerns. She was so bright and full of life. I was terribly afraid our separations would scar her for life, turning her into a child lacking confidence and happiness. I knew Mom wouldn't spoil her and would demand good behavior even if life was upside-down. Consistency was non-existent in much of our lives; yet we had to strive for it as much as possible.

On Monday, Richmond, Kyle and I drove to Stanford. Surgery, however, was canceled that day. The next day—again no surgery, just another needle biopsy, and no clear explanation why. We went for lunch at the Stanford Mall and did some "therapy shopping," wandering around looking for nothing in particular. We hoped an appointment with the doctors would clear up our confusion about why the surgery was canceled, but for now we waited, and waited, to hear what the program would be. We found ourselves talking about anything but Kyle's cancer. Speculating—when we had so little information—was not how we wanted to spend time. It was easier to stay away from a subject so intensely emotional, when we knew there would be plenty of time for serious discussions later. My mind fought off the idea that our baby could die from cancer; my lips would not even let the words pass.

That day, Richmond and I took Kyle to a meeting room where Dr. Mogul, Dr. Gary Dahl and the family therapist waited to discuss Kyle's upcoming protocol. Dr. Dahl was tall and thin with dark hair, and a warm smile that immediately made us feel more at ease. He and Dr. Mogul made a good team. They told us Kyle's surgery had been canceled because the tumor entwined his intestines and required shrinking with chemo before removal was possible.

There were papers to sign, and right at the top of the first page it read:

"Experimental Subject Agreement"

Boy, they didn't sugarcoat anything. No hidden meaning there. This was an experiment and Kyle was subject No. 100 in the study. The 100 kids were from all over the country and would be on the exact same protocol: five rounds of chemotherapy. Days One through Seven meant Cytoxan, given orally by us at home. Day Eight was an IV of Adriamycin. The next three weeks, Kyle was to recover from chemo, and on Day 28 he would start over again.

His therapy would continue on schedule, provided his blood counts recovered to an acceptable level. Chemo identifies and kills all the fastest-growing cells in the body. Hair follicles, gastrointestinal tract, bone marrow and tumor cells are at the top of the "hit list." The gastro-tract is your mouth all the way down to your rear end. The blood counts also go way down—often to near nothing. Red blood cells—hemoglobin—need to be greater than 8.0, or a transfusion is necessary. Platelets have to be greater than 15, or again, a transfusion is necessary. Neutrophils are the greater portion of all white blood cells, and their number fits into an equation called the absolute neutophil count (ANC). The ANC must be greater than 500 to start a new round of chemotherapy. These blood counts are significantly lower than what's expected in a healthy individual.

After five rounds of chemo, the doctors expected to remove what was left of the tumor, maybe proceed with some more chemo—and that would be that. Being an optimist, that sounded pretty good to me. A little chemo, maybe his hair would fall out, a little surgery, and see ya later!

Still, I was very confused, and so was Richmond. Nature Boy, of course, wanted to know what else we could do. The thought of this chemotherapy regimen totally went against his grain. Chemo killed *all* fast-growing cells. This sounded really bad in a baby, since all his cells were growing so fast. The doctors reassured us and explained that it was our only choice. Well, that certainly narrowed it down. Dr. Mogul explained again that the fastest-growing cells in our bodies are our hair follicles, the gastro-tract, the bone marrow and cancer cells. That is why there are a lot of bald people throwing up in cancer wards. As soon as chemo is stopped, the cells grow back fast, except (hopefully) the cancerous ones. That is the theory behind chemotherapy.

I thought I should ask more questions, but I was at a loss. One question in particular dogged Richmond and me: Why did our baby get cancer? Was it something I'd eaten or drunk while pregnant? Was it the chemicals I'd worked with as a roofer? Richmond asked if it was genetic. *Anything* would help, if we just knew why! Not knowing was awful.

Dr. Mogul replied, "Check guilt off your list. We just don't know what causes this disease. If we knew, we would have the Nobel Prize in medicine."

That was valuable advice. We would never know why Kyle had neuroblastoma. All we knew was it was a nerve cell tumor. People used to ask me, "What is neuroblastoma?" My reply: "It's a blast of nerves. A bunch of nerve cells had a party and it got way out of hand."

Now all we had to do was get started to put an end to this party.

That evening, Kyle was given his first dose of Cytoxan. Our regular nurse wasn't allowed to administer it because she was pregnant. That drove home how toxic the drug was. Another nurse brought in a clear syringe (without a needle) to administer the clear liquid Cytoxan. She squirted it in Kyle's mouth a little at a time. As she gave him his first dose, he squirmed and made a face indicating serious distaste. He had to be held down, one hand holding his head stationary, so he wouldn't spit out any of the drug. With the drug administered, our nurse was on her way to her next task.

Kyle and I were starting to get settled into Children's. This was starting to feel OK. I went to the women's room, which was shared by all the parents and patients, to freshen up. Quite the busy place! There sat Kendra. Her mom was cutting her hair. Or should I say whacking it off—and with paper scissors, no less. I'm thinking, *Gee, nice 'do*. I felt like such an idiot when I realized that all her hair was falling out, anyway. This would simply minimize the hassle.

The next morning I was walking down the corridor. I looked in Kendra's room and saw her holding something I couldn't quite identify. She and her roommate were laughing like a couple of schoolgirls.

"What is that, Kendra?" I asked. "It looks like a coconut."

"Oh this?" she said laughing. "It's a hairball. You should have seen the residents' faces. It really freaked them out."

This was followed by more laughter as she and her roommate had really gotten one over on the new residents.

Kendra then offered a practical explanation. "I just got tired of going to the wastebasket. My hair is falling out so fast."

I couldn't imagine anything worse for a 15-year-old girl. How much time did they spend on their hair everyday? She must have felt like hiding, but she didn't. Kendra met everything head on. That was her style.

Wednesday was Richmond's and my third wedding anniversary. But our thoughts were consumed with Kyle's low hemoglobin count, 6.8. A blood transfusion was scheduled.

A transfusion? Does he really need one? The nurses were polite and didn't point out the obvious—Kyle was very pale. Darn it, that hemoglobin was handy for keeping color in his cheeks. Richmond and Anna had driven in from Reno to join us. Richmond asked if he could donate and was told yes, but the blood had to be irradiated, which took hours. Kyle needed a transfusion immediately. Richmond was told who to go through to arrange a donation for future use. Kyle's blood was B+ and he also required CMV negative blood. CMV is a virus that 97 percent of the population has at some time in their lives. The virus never leaves a person's system once infected. So he needed B+, CMV negative, irradiated blood.

This was all getting so complicated. Little did we know that transfusions were passed out here like hamburgers at a fast-food joint.

But we were learning this cancer ward game.

My Brother is
on the bed.
he is geting
a ball out of
his chast

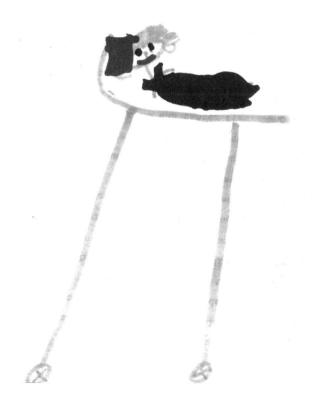

CHAPTER 3

WELCOME TO THE CHEMO CLUB

It was now apparent that not only would we be at Stanford a lot, but quite a bit of our time might be spent in outpatient care. Richmond was a wonderful provider, but the Hyatt wasn't in our budget! We sat down to ponder our options.

Richmond had a friend who lived near Stanford and was a resident physician in the neurosurgery program. Kim Page Stone was an ambitious woman in her mid thirties, with straight sandy-brown hair, a terrific figure and comforting smile. She had recently married another surgeon who was on the teaching staff at Stanford Medical Center. His name was Jim Stone. I had met Kim once at a party her father threw for her when she was accepted into the neurosurgery program. It had been a few years, but I remember I'd really liked her. Richmond had roomed with her in college along with another student. Neither of us had met her husband.

Richmond called Kim and started explaining our situation. She was stunned. It turned out she had been standing in the hallway about 15 feet from me when Dr. Hartman had told me he was 90 percent sure Kyle had neuroblastoma. We hadn't recognized each other. Kim later told me that she had been thinking, "that poor mom," and it had felt almost dream-like. What a small world.

Kim and Jim opened their home to us. A pretty brave move! We met them on their doorstep. Jim, also in his thirties, was athletic with curly brown hair and a great sense of humor.

Their generosity was overwhelming. And while it felt very weird staying at someone else's house, all in all the situation was a godsend. The Stones had a very nice home just a short distance from the hospital. Jim had an extensive background in oncology. The entire combination was too good to be true. Wonderful friends that were close to the hospital, and with medical knowledge. Their medical background was an added plus. It waved the task of explaining about Kyle's condition. I had already spent a lot of time and energy trying to make those around me feel better about Kyle. I had to tell people we were doing fine, when we weren't. After all, what's "fine" in the cancer world is frightening in the real world.

Kim and Jim knew exactly what every procedure, test and result meant. They didn't greet us with fear of the unknown or sadness. Each daily drama for Kyle and me was just another day for them in their business. That helped keep me going. They were extremely compassionate, too—and also very busy. That meant I often had time to myself in their very beautiful home. Time to regroup and gather myself.

I often cooked dinner for Kim and Jim when Kyle and I stayed over. They had such hectic schedules that home-cooked meals were not an everyday occurrence for them. I pitched in whenever my schedule allowed.

Before long, Kim and I would tease Jim that he had two wives. He would walk through the door to the smell of dinner cooking. I would greet him with a grin, "Hi honey, welcome home." It would give us all a good laugh. This adopted home life was wonderful for Kyle and me; and Richmond had peace of mind knowing his wife and son were living somewhere safe. There were times I wondered what would have happened to us if we hadn't had that safety net. The local Ronald McDonald House—the clean, $10-a-night haven for families of cancer patients—was over-booked due to remodeling. Meanwhile, the lower-priced hotels left much to be desired, and the Stanford area was not cheap. Kyle and I might have ended up sleeping in our Suburban truck (indeed, Richmond did a couple of nights in the early going). I knew people who brought motorhomes to the back parking lot at Children's. It was a real consideration.

As luck would have it, Kim and Jim usually had room for us during our Stanford visits. A true gift!

Richmond went back to Reno while Kyle finished chemo. We went in for outpatient chemo. I had never been in a do-or-die situation. Literally! If Kyle didn't take his chemo—that was it. Taking the drugs wasn't easy for a baby. Chemo wasn't fruit-flavored like other children's medicine. Kyle would cringe and squirm during the administration of each dose, indicating the taste was foul. Chemo was far too toxic to do a taste check. The tension ran high, and I felt a tremendous relief after each dose had been successfully administered.

Friday 9/28/90
Blood work looks good. Chemo has gone well all week. Driving home, in Davis, CA., supra pubic tube falls out of Kyle's abdomen. Drive 3 hours back to Stanford. Tube is reinserted. I am not completely convinced that there isn't anything left behind in his bladder. BAD DAY! Stay at Kim and Jim's.

That Friday was the only time I had felt that our crisis wasn't fair, and I verbally screamed this many times. Kyle and I pulled into Davis. I changed his diaper on a blanket on a lawn next to the parking lot, as usual. When I saw the tube fall out, I just fell apart.

I stood over Kyle nearly hysterical and cried out, "Oh my God, Oh my God. No! This can't be happening. Oh my God!"

A young woman with a small child in a stroller happened to be walking by. She quickly came over and asked if she could help.

I blurted, "My baby has cancer and this tube just fell out of him. Can you watch him? I have to call his doctor immediately!"

That poor woman didn't know what to say except, "Of course."

I had never done anything remotely close to leaving my baby attended by a total stranger. But I figured hearing what she heard, even if she were a baby kidnapper, he wouldn't have been a good candidate. I ran across the short parking lot shaded with trees to the pay phone. Crying as I rummaged for change, my emotions veered from anger to fear and back again. I reached the doctors. Finding I had to return to Stanford left me wilted with anguish. I called Mom in Reno to notify her of the situation, then returned to where Kyle lay. The young woman stood by him with her baby still in the stroller.

"Is there anything else I can do to help?" she said.

"No, thank you for helping," I replied, sobbing. "Making that call was what I needed to do. Now we have to go back to get the tube put back in."

The woman looked at me with kind eyes, and turned to leave. Then she paused. "I was having a bad day up until now and feeling pretty sorry for myself," she said. "Thanks for putting my life into perspective."

The hospital told me to come back and they would take care of Kyle. To add insult to injury, I knew rush-hour traffic in San Francisco on a Friday afternoon would be excruciating. It was.

I had already called home earlier to tell Mom, Anna and Richmond I was on my way. Anna told Mom she didn't believe I was coming back. I understood. Everything about our lives was so uncertain then. To have to call back and tell them I really wasn't coming was one of the worst moments of my life. I cried and screamed, "It's not fair!" all the way back to Stanford.

I felt so awful for Anna. She was old enough to know what was going on and she didn't like it. The rest of us didn't like it either, but at least we knew what the program would be, and we were as mentally prepared as anyone could have been. Kyle himself was fairly unaffected. At 4 months old, a lot of his program was nursing and sleeping. He didn't seem particular where he did it.

Saturday morning, Kyle and I drove home, for a respite of only a day and a half before we would have to return to Stanford. Richmond, Mom and I decided Anna needed to be with me no matter where we were, so Mom, Anna, Kyle and I drove back to Stanford for Kyle's IV of Adriamycin chemotherapy. Thursday, a few days after Kyle had completed the Adriamycin, I could hear a strange raspiness in his voice. I finally connected it with the chemo. His gastro-tract was raw and would recover soon. It made me cry that I could even hear the damage to his poor little body. But I considered that so far, Kyle hadn't thrown up. He was nursing well, had just had his first baby rice cereal and was in really great spirits. If this was as bad as it would get, we were going to get through it.

Then that Monday, he threw up four times, and could only keep down two meals. Tuesday, he threw up twice. Dr. Mogul said if that was his worst reaction, he was doing fine. Well, maybe things weren't going to be quite that easy. Before long, I decided to burp Kyle over the sink. He was throwing up after feedings quite often. It didn't take a rocket scientist to figure out why. Chemotherapy is so hard on the stomach (part of the gastro-tract) that nausea is the norm, often accompanied with by vomiting. Aside from this, things seemed all right. We had some days at home as a family. We really came to appreciate our time together. I would look at my husband and thank God that we had each other. Anna was especially helpful in keeping us grounded. I knew Richmond would do

OK, but there was a 2-year-old that still needed a sandwich for lunch, a nap, books read to her. Anna's demands meant there wasn't any time to fall apart. Life had to go on—and did.

There were times I forgot that Richmond would need my support, also. When the stress and fear became too much, he would grow crabby, then identify the reason and ultimately break down and cry. It seemed to work out well. Our "break down" days always seemed to alternate, with one of us falling apart and the other staying strong. Many days we were both strong and enjoying life. There were a few days here and there to regroup between trips to the hospital. We spent a lot of time hugging and just doing regular daily activities. I put my membership to the gym on hold, because I only spent time in three places: the hospital, home, or the grocery store. I still liked preparing gourmet meals, and we all really enjoyed them. It was an activity that brought us all together.

I found that I saw the gas station attendants in Davis (my halfway point on the commute) and Stanford more than many of our good friends. Even the bagel and coffee guy at the coffeehouse I stopped at in Davis would inquire about Kyle. An odd network of acquaintances had formed. Ironically, a number of our friends were afraid to call. Some were fearful of what they might hear, or worried that they would be "bothering" us. Cancer has a way of casting a blanket of dread over many hearts. I know our friends cared and many did call, but fear does funny things to people. One of our friends who was working with Richmond at the time had seen his mother die of cancer. He was candid in disclosing his feelings.

"I'm sorry, I just can't get close," he said. "It's not that I don't care, but I won't be asking. I just can't handle it. I'm sorry, but I won't be much help."

I admired his honesty. It took a lot of courage for him to say that.

Many people who did call would only ask about Kyle. Of course, that was understandable. But I got so tired of people forgetting to ask about Anna that sometimes I would say, "Oh yeah, Anna's doing fine." After all, she would be sitting there playing and knew exactly what was going on. I tried to keep her in focus as much as I could. Thank God, Richmond was so dedicated to our daughter. With her interest in mind, Richmond and I kept our family life as normal as possible. Thus, we consulted Dr. Colletti, our pediatrician, about keeping Round 2 of chemo at a nearby hospital. He agreed, wrote the prescription for seven days of Cytoxan and made an appointment at Saint Mary's, one of the two local hospitals, for the IV of Adriamycin on Day Eight.

Giving Kyle his doses of Cytoxan was a serious challenge. Anna demanded a lot of attention as does any 2-year-old, and often at inappropriate times—such as when Kyle needed his chemo. Richmond and I worked together holding Kyle and giving him a syringe of liquid chemo orally. He would writhe and fuss, making faces communicating that it tasted like poison. In a real sense it was poison, though it served its purpose. After that, antibiotics or any medicines were no big deal for him. The 10 minutes it took to give Kyle his chemo felt like an hour, and you could have cut the tension in the air with a knife. We knew that his only chance for survival was chemo, regardless of our fears associated with such a strong drug. We got through each dose and went on with the day trying to shake off the stress.

THE DAYS PASSED, AND the holiday season neared. I knew Anna had to go trick-or-treating. Like it or not, I had to get some costumes together for the kids.

Richmond is a hunter and we had a surplus of buckskin from deer. The Halloween costumes for Anna and Kyle would be fashioned out of buckskin. Kyle already had little moccasins. I cut out vests for both kids and a wrap-around skirt for Anna. They all had ties that kept them together, and fringe on the bottom. Then we made head-dresses for both. Richmond had feathers from hunting, so Anna set the feathers in glue on a long strip of buckskin for both Kyle and herself and I topped them with another strip. The two looked adorable as little Indians.

Kyle's IV of Adriamycin came on Halloween, also. "Gotta have a good time," was our motto, so I took him in full costume for his chemo. The nurses were pleasantly surprised and we all got quite a few laughs out of our approach to cancer therapy. In Reno, there wasn't a pediatric oncology unit, so the nurses weren't as used to the humor that I had developed at Stanford. At Stanford, most of the kids wore their costumes, because, cancer or not—holidays continue, life goes on, and it's best that way.

The frequency of IV starts became a real problem for me and Kyle. His tiny veins were hard to hit. When I would phone Stanford Children's Hospital to tell them we were coming, they would make calls to all the different units to find out who the best IV starter was. We didn't even mind the IVs anymore, as long as they could get it going in one, two or three tries. For many months, I would hold Kyle flat on a table while a nurse would try for an IV insertion. He was so little that it was nice to be able to hold him the second they were done. I also wanted to help with his care. Sometimes it took six or seven tries. I knew medicine was not an exact science, and I also knew that these people were doing a job so terribly difficult that most people couldn't stand it for a week. They were the cream of the crop. Kyle was just a hard poke. And that wasn't the end of his problems.

With each passing week, Kyle was becoming more and more sick. Throwing up was not that big of a deal. We were worried about death. Was the chemo working? We didn't care about the nausea as long as we felt the chemo was worth it. Tests, tests, and more tests. We were beginning to understand what they were all for and what the results meant. We always asked. Fortunately, the doctors always took the time to answer.

On Nov. 7, we got the news. The tumor had shrunk. I could hardly believe it! In one short sentence the doctors had given us incredible hope. I was amazed by the feeling that came over me. It was as if heavy stones had been lifted from my shoulders. I started crying and couldn't stop, feeling as though I would collapse. It took nearly 30 minutes to slow my tears of relief and joy. Walking down the hallway to use the Teddy Bear Phone, I passed people who looked afraid to ask why I was crying.

I was barely able to calm myself as Richmond answered the phone. He could hear I had been crying. He braced himself for the worst. He felt the same relief that I did upon hearing the news. It was our first milestone on the road to success. We hoped we would reach others. We were confident we would.

I should say that through all this, the insurance company had been wonderful. What?! Yes, wonderful. It never missed a beat, paid on time, and never flinched at the astronomical bills we were accumulating. Thank God I had signed with it for our health care. Our insurance agent had recommended this company because it was respectable and paid on time. My late step-father had been an insurance agent and always said, "Go with someone that pays on time." At least that wasn't a worry. We had enough worries.

Blood work was a daily routine in the hospital for us now, including before and after many tests. Kyle kept his happy-go-lucky attitude through each session of jabbing and poking, and returned to "Smiley Kyley" as soon as they stopped bugging him.

On Nov. 8, Kyle ran his first serious fever—100.4. His blood counts were very low when his fever came and IV antibiotics were needed. He suffered from neutropenia—a blood count that is very low in neutrophils. Everyone needs these cells, which make up the majority of white blood cells. I used to call them, "puny neutros," when there weren't enough for a good count. The condition is also called "F&N"—fever and neutropenia. This was all news to me as I had never known anything about blood work. The fever Kyle had would almost go unnoticed on any other child. Under normal circumstances, a Children's Tylenol and popsicle would probably be a sufficient cure, not IV antibiotics for five to 10 days. It was almost unbelievable.

My journal reveals Kyle's medication for F&N:

11/8/90
IV Antibiotics

1. Fluconozole

2. Nafcillin   4 times a day

3. Azlocillin   4 times a day

4. Amikacin   3 times a day

Check blood levels every day before administering.

Wow! That was certainly no popsicle and Tylenol. I was stunned upon realizing the significance of a low ANC (absolute neutrophil count). What's "low" in the cancer world is "desperately, frighteningly low" in the rest of the world. A normal ANC can be around 5,000, whereas Kyle's counts went to 0 on a number of occasions. Of course, I was new at this, so I barely had a clue, anyway.

The next day, his ANC fell to 28. It needed to be at 500 for us to go home. By now I was used to roadblocks on the way to recovery. My journal entries noted:

Personal 11/9/90
It has been almost 2 mo. since Kyle's diagnosis, and now is

our first time we are in for a fever. His ANC is 28 today, was 180 yesterday, and needs to be 500 to go home. It's kind of a drag, but we do the best we can. I am in a room right now with a 4 year old girl with A.L.L., a kind of Leukemia, Alena's little boy, with I don't know what, and a little Mexican girl who's not yet diagnosed, and they don't even speak English.

Alena and I went to Pedro's and had a few beers. It was a great relief after being in here all day except 20 minutes. Tomorrow Richmond and Anna come to visit. Thank God! With his counts this way, it could be weeks before we get out of here. Maybe not.

Pedro's, the local Mexican restaurant and cantina at Stanford Mall, became our "Parent Therapy" center. It was about 1,000 paces from the hospital door. Alaska Bob (Cassie's dad and our first roommate), would go, along with Alena and a few other parents. The nurses would give us a beeper that they could call us on if one of our kids woke up and couldn't be consoled. Pedro's offered a great way to shake off the hospital and get some hearty laughs. Laughter was a potent release, and we could all make bad jokes about things we'd seen or heard in the hospital. After the kids were asleep for the night we would wander over to Pedro's and almost feel like normal people again. Some of our humor brought sideways glances from customers who were certain they couldn't have heard us correctly. We had a lot of material to work with: kids throwing up constantly; the doctors and nurses; who was in the ward; who went home; and the comments that the kids made.

The kids were unreal, measuring hair or lack thereof. Kyle only had three eyelashes per eye; it looked like someone had been gluing them on him when the phone rang and the job never finished. Kyle never stopped smiling. A doctor came in one morning just to say, "hi," though he wasn't even Kyle's doctor. Kyle smiled at him, threw up, and smiled again. The doctor just tossed up his arms and said, "That's it! I can't believe how happy this kid is!" He was not alone in this sentiment.

Kyle and I played baby games as he lay in his metal crib, in a constant effort to keep him from pulling on "the great tube" that was always there. Those IV tubes were terrific entertainment for a little one. He just kept smiling no matter what happened. Kyle's attitude was such an incredible blessing. I couldn't imagine what it would have been like if he had been a cranky baby by nature. His constant gurgles and smiles kept me going.

Waiting for the Teddy Bear Phone was often a time-consuming event. Sometimes the line was long. Once in awhile it was free when I showed up. The house rule was a 10-minute limit, but if no one was there you could talk as long as you wanted. I was so thankful that service was provided. When I was down at Stanford, having spent many hours, then days, with no reprieve, the phone was my life-line. Having a tie to the outside world was a true blessing. The waits could be lengthy, though. Not good at being sedentary, I had already decided that exercising whenever possible would be a bonus. Sometimes I would do jumping jacks while waiting for the Teddy Bear Phone. Of course, the others teased me, so I just said, "You should all get off your butts and do something while you wait."

One morning, three or four of us were all doing jumping jacks, sit-ups and toe-touches. Our "aerobics class" had no music, hardly any room, and participants were constantly leaving to use the phone. Hospital personnel of one kind or another walked through the hall and must have been sure that we were parents who had lost it. My motto was, "Gotta have a Good Time." Stand and wait may have been the rule of thumb, but I wasn't good at that. I ran everywhere I went and was probably lucky I hadn't creamed anybody in a hallway. The old Children's Hospital at Stanford was one story, spread out, with lots of crossing halls. People would say as I ran, "Is everything OK?" I would reply, "I just like to run." In actuality, I didn't like to run, but it was something I could do for exercise at the hospital, on the grounds, or on "field trips" with Kyle.

Any available entertainment was a plus. The hospital had a library for patients and parents. One of the things on the list to check out was a video camera. I had never operated one, but thought it would be a gas to make a home movie. For one thing, no one knew what we did all day, every day. Even Richmond hadn't spent a whole lot of time at the hospital. I was definitely the hospital parent. I actually kind of liked it there when I was immersed in it. When I was "living" at the hospital it became the "norm." As soon as I stepped out of that world, though, my God! What a bizarre existence it seemed. However, I had developed a circle of friends at the hospital and felt it would be fun to have a home movie with them in it.

The video camera was broken and would not be repaired for weeks. In the meantime, I began developing my movie ideas, and constantly checked on the camera's status. I had always had the drive to document the moment at hand; and hospital life was no different. It wasn't the typical family scene, but I felt every bit as worthy of chronicling, if not more so. I wanted people in my family to "meet" all the great people at the hospital. There were so many who were not only caregivers, but truly felt like friends.

I outlined my ideas in my journal:

World Famous Oncologist Dr. Mark Mogul

Aerobics in Phone line

Transport Team

Day Hospital

Rollo Singing

Pedro's—Parent Therapy

The nurses at any hospital are busy, busy, busy! At the children's cancer ward they were jammin'! This explains the following anecdote. Kyle's supra pubic tube was located about 2 inches above his belly button. The site looked quite a bit like an "inny," and if you weren't looking real close you would have thought it was a second belly button.

I was always a participating parent, and one afternoon upon returning from lunch, I went to check to see if Kyle needed a dry diaper. His supra pubic tube still required a little antibiotic cream and a bandage. No big deal!

As I opened the diaper to check the status, I started laughing my head off! His belly button had ointment and a patch on it. I had to call in the nurse, because I wanted her to get a chuckle too.

"What can I do for you?" she inquired, as she walked into the room.

"You have to see this," I replied laughing. "It's too funny. Someone patched his belly button."

"Oh," she replied embarrassed. "I didn't do that."

"Yeah." I teased. "Sure you didn't."

As she walked back out of the room, I chuckled, enjoying the humor.

Kyle was improving. Even the rash on his butt was going away thanks to balm. On Nov. 13, we were heading home.

Going home! There was an amazing amount of happiness in simply pulling up in the truck in front of our house. I could no longer understand how people could bitch about a dent in their car or all the other things that are small stuff. We learned that lesson in a big way. I managed to gear up for the hospital runs, almost pretending that we were going to the park. After all, the doctors had a plan. They didn't just shake our hands and say, "I'm sorry." So went my program. *Forward with the plan.* Thank God for the new friends, and the chemo we hoped would cure Kyle.

It finally dawned on me that I also needed to "gear up" to go home. We were a family. I couldn't just drive in, drop Kyle, and get pampered. The nightmare never quit running, and though it was a different location, we still had to work together. I began to formulate the game plan for going home. What would Richmond like for dinner the next evening? Was there any food in the house? Did the laundry need to be done?

Richmond was doing a great job on the home front. Business was good. Clients were happy and the money kept coming in. Anna was surrounded by people who loved her. My stepmother, Leigh, Richmond's sister, Debbie, and my Mom were all tremendous caregivers for our little daughter. We were a family who all pitched in to help. I realized at that point that Anna, Richmond, Kyle and I all "deserved a vote." Kyle was the only one with cancer, but we all counted. We had to make sure that we all had some recovery time.

Our lives were on hold from that standpoint, because all our "free time" was spent restoring energy, talking to each other and hugging. We needed to get grounded every chance we could.

CHAPTER 4

THE HOLIDAYS

When I was younger and would complain about something insignificant, my Mom would say, "If you think you have problems, go down to a cancer ward, you'll see people with real problems." She probably doesn't say that anymore, but she was correct, and taught me to hold onto that viewpoint. She always looked for the good. If one could stay tough yet ride the rainbow, life would be grand. And it was.

We were starting Round 3 of chemo. It hadn't been easy, but we were holding up well. The side-effects we were warned about were present. Kyle was bald as could be. Not a hair was left on his little head, and only three eyelashes remained on each eye. Even facial fuzz was gone. He threw up a lot during the week that his counts were low, but his zest for life continued. We remained optimistic. After all, the doctors had tossed us a bone—the medicine was working. The tumor had shrunk.

After the terrible stress of giving Kyle chemo orally at home, we were looking for an alternative. The liquid Cytoxan was clear and looked the same as baby drool, thus we were expending way too much energy worrying if he was taking all of it. Dr. Mogul suggested crushing a tablet in some of his favorite food. Richmond thought bananas might work. Great idea! I would laugh a witch's cackle and tease, "Here, little boy, have some poison bananas." It was easy to laugh. The bananas worked like a charm. The relief was incredible, and Kyle didn't seem to mind at all.

Thankful was an understatement for that year's Thanksgiving holiday. We were together as a family. Kyle's treatments were progressing in a positive direction, and the rest of us were healthy. Just being at the same table breaking bread brought tears of joy to many an eye.

Every day held a question mark. Where would Kyle and Donna be? Reno or Palo Alto? The lack of concrete planning in our lives was something we were becoming used to.

One social aspect of our lives that we missed was having friends over to dinner. Richmond and I both loved to cook and entertain. He was fabulous at preparing creative meals and though I did the bulk of it, he would always pitch in. At that point in our lives, just getting dinner on the table was an accomplishment. At times I felt so isolated. I had no social life, though I had lots of support from friends and family. It wasn't the same as simply going out to lunch with a girlfriend.

I felt really lucky to have made all the new friends among hospital personnel. The people I met at Children's Hospital at Stanford were compassionate, wonderful human beings. They had to be. Working in a cancer ward takes a unique kind of person, from the friendly woman that I saw keeping the floors immaculate to the doctors handing orders to the nurses. One of the requirements is a heart about four sizes too big and a smile that is always available.

Kyle had trouble with IV starts everywhere, but in Reno we had a more difficult time. Kyle's veins were so scarred at the ripe age of 6 months that he was a very difficult poke. The Reno caregivers were qualified and compassionate, but the regular pediatric ward was considerably different from a pediatric oncology ward. A cancer ward has a different mindset, with life and death a daily, even hourly, issue. Most pediatric floors are considerably more low-key. I was glad that I was so involved in Kyle's health care, because I knew what to ask, and what many of the answers meant.

When working with the local hospital, we were very happy with Dr. Colletti, our pediatrician. He was supportive and compassionate, and had already shown his true colors in the heat of battle. He was terrific. We wanted to do some of the chemo locally and Dr. Colletti had said he would help with the treatment if it was Group A of the chemo drugs. He had seen the protocol sheets and did not want to work with Group B, whose possible side effects were kidney damage, hearing loss and required hospitalization prior to administering the doses, for pre-hydration. The drugs and side effects were more serious, and we had always admired his honesty.

I was becoming an old hand at this business. Kyle's blood count on Nov. 30 showed his platelets down to 20, and white blood cell count at 1.0. He underwent a platelet transfusion that day and again on Dec. 2. The CBC (complete blood count) showed platelets only up to 21, hemoglobin at 8.5 and white blood count at 0.6. I called Dr. Mogul, who said it was OK to take Kyle home if the platelets count was greater than 15 and the hemoglobin count was greater than 8.0.

That was the only time I checked Kyle out of a hospital on my own accord. I knew what blood levels were acceptable. Dr. Colletti wasn't on call, and the doctor present wasn't familiar enough with our case to make me happy. In the "real world" Kyle's counts threw up all the red flags, but in the cancer world these were everyday counts, expected and not alarming.

The nurses at Saint Mary's knew I was fully informed about my son's health care. I asked for the chart, looked at the blood counts, and knew what had to be done. They just weren't used to these drastically low numbers. We could walk into the lab on any day of the week at that point and have a CBC (complete blood count) done. There was a standing order from Dr. Colletti with the local blood lab. If Kyle's hemoglobin or platelet count proved to be too low I would either call Dr. Colletti or Dr. Mogul, depending on where we wanted to get the transfusion.

It got to the point where, on a given day, I could pull Kyle's eyelid down and, by looking at the degree of redness, come close to guessing his hemoglobin number. When I went into the Saint Mary's lab, I would say, "Hi" to the gal running the desk ordering blood work, and tell her what I thought his number would be. There were a few days I hit it right on the head. It was a game of sorts, and helped keep interest and humor in our lives. The platelets weren't anything I could guess. All I knew was they kept you from bleeding to death. I always drove with extra caution when Kyle's platelet count was really low, knowing a car wreck could bring an injury with unstoppable bleeding.

12/3/90 Medical
*St. Mary's-platelet count—3. May Day! All Kyle's veins have
been blown out. Surgeon must put IV into large vein in Kyle's
neck. chloral hydrate (sleep) and xylocaine to numb area.
Kyle MUST have platelets.*

12/3/90 Personal
*It's been a long week. It's been a long fall. We are surviving
and doing well on some days and falling apart on some days.
The last week we've been in/out/in/out and back again. I am
stenciling a red poinsettia with paint on all our Christmas
envelopes and letters tonight.*

That visit to the local hospital proved far more complicated
than we had bargained for. All Kyle's veins were blown and he
was unbelievably low on platelets. Seeing the surgeon cut into
Kyle's neck was almost more than I could take. I felt so very helpless and frightened. They had poked, then poked again and again.
Then they had made an incision. I wanted to scream. I began to
cry. I was feeling incredibly worn down and vulnerable. Richmond
was a wonderful support, but we both felt strongly that Anna
needed him there and my place was with Kyle. We would be
together to rejuvenate whenever possible. He had always said
whenever I needed him he would be there.

There were days when I said out loud to myself, "Oh my God—
I just can't take this." But I did, and found that after a "breakdown
day" I would have new energy to hit our challenges head on. I had
also found a pattern to my coping. On Day Five of heavy hospital
work, I would always need a good cry. Those first four days I could
do *anything*—no problem. On the fifth day it was as if a heavy
blanket covered my body, accompanied by a numbness. The cure
seemed to be a serious sob session. Occasionally, someone would
notice the puffy red eyes and ask if I was OK. "I'm OK. This is just
my breakdown day," I would reply. "Tomorrow I'll be better."

And so the cycle went.

At that point, my patience level was about as low as it could
get. I made a decision that all Kyle's health care would be at
Children's Hospital at Stanford—period. The five-hour drive was
worth the peace of mind, so I called Dr. Mogul and let him know
we needed to find an alternative. He said that when Kyle spiked a
fever with low counts, traveling five hours with no antibiotics was

too long to wait. If and when he had F&N again, we would have to go to the emergency room (ER) and get 500 milligrams of ceftriaxone (split 250 mg per thigh).

A few days later, Kyle spiked a fever at 4 a.m. Up we got, dressed, hunk of toast, cup of joe and off for the blood work. It just amazed me that five hours was too long to wait for a medication when his counts were so low. In the "old days," if Anna had a fever I never thought a whole lot about it. I certainly didn't run to the ER and the lab. Now we were in another world.

I'll never forget the Saint Mary's ER that morning in Reno. I went in and told the nurses we needed a blood draw. "My son has cancer," I said. "He has spiked a fever, and depending on his counts, he'll need IV antibiotics as soon as possible." The whole statement left the staff a bit shaken. They weren't accustomed to that kind of statement coming from a parent.

Kyle's blood was drawn and we waited for the counts. When they came back, they were given to the pediatrician on call. She could have used a refresher course in Bedside 101. I told her what the scoop was. She relayed that his counts were low, so I passed on the prescription: "500 milligrams ceftriaxone split intramuscularly." She took one look at me, like, who the hell did I think I was?! So I gave her Dr. Mogul's beeper number and told her to call him. He reiterated my orders and she quickly took care of us.

Off to ER we went, where the pediatrician had called in the order. The guy in ER was so stunned at the amount of ceftriaxone ordered for this baby that he "suggested" he double-check with Kyle's oncologist. I said, "Fine with me, just get on it!" He came back a moment later, and asked us to come on back for the shots.

Afterward, we went home and grabbed our bags. They were always packed for a journey. I had learned that we could be gone for two days, or two weeks. I never knew what Kyle's counts would be. At a certain point, his body would start to recover from the chemo and counts might start doubling everyday. Sometimes they would hit a low and it seemed to really drag. Upon returning from each trip, I would remove all the dirty clothes, replenish the bags with clean clothes, and refill all shampoo and conditioner containers, and so on. This method worked well, considering fever and neutropenia knew no hours and had little consideration. If our bags happened to be empty, I could pack for a two-week stay in about 10 minutes. I had always been organized and this was a time in my life when this virtue really came in handy.

Up until this point, I had a lot of naiveté left in me. I figured if Kyle took his medicine and the experts said his chances were good, pretty much that was that. No big deal. Kyle would get sick, go bald and our lives would be a wreck for awhile, but he would live. This overall view was seriously altered one day at Stanford.

Walking down the hallway, wasting time, I stopped to glance at the bulletin board by the clinic. There was an article posted about a young woman of 16 who had recently died of cancer. It told of glorious things that her school, friends and family had planned for her because they knew she was going to die. The events had been rewarding for everyone involved. It hit me like a ton of bricks. I had met this young woman, though only briefly, when she was Kendra's roommate. I knew who her mother was, but had never spoken to her. I'd always wondered why the mother looked so unhappy. How could I have been so stupid?! Her daughter was dying. I was stunned. This girl was the first person at the hospital I'd met who had died. It scared the hell out of me. I fully realized, at that moment, that they didn't all make it out alive.

I checked in at the nurses' station and left the hospital grounds. I started wandering, in a stupor. My revelation changed everything. I started saying prayers for the girl's family and mine. The whole situation left me amazed that I could have been so naive.

The big picture looked different now. When I looked in people's faces, it wasn't for a superficial smile, or greeting. The body language of each told a different story, and I knew then that even though there were always question marks, our prognosis was good, and there were many who couldn't say the same. Mom's survivalist attitude stayed with me: "If you think you have problems, look around." She would have never said that to me at that point, but it was still valid. Perhaps more than ever.

We were on our way to Round 4 of chemo. It was to conclude on Christmas Eve, with Richmond, Anna, Kyle and me returning to our home that evening. There were always more tests to see how things were progressing. One of the critical tests was a bone marrow "aspiration." Dr. Mogul took a big fat needle, stuck it into Kyle's pelvic bone from the backside, and sucked out marrow. Even under sedation, Kyle squirmed and whimpered. If the bone marrow had cancer in it—the whole picture would be changed.

Thank God, the test results were clear.

We still had many friends and family members who weren't even remotely aware of what was going on with us and Kyle's cancer, so we decided to send out a Christmas letter:

Hello and Seasons Greetings,

What a year it has been! We haven't spoken with or seen many of you for too long! We miss seeing and talking to your smiling faces, and hope 1990 was a great year for you. I'm sure if we were together now, sitting by a warm fire, sipping a steaming cup of brew, we could share some fine stories and tell tales of great adventures. And in our hearts we are. So perhaps you should grab a mug of your favorite libation, nestle in by a warm fire, and we'll tell you a story about our lives this year.

The first five months of 1990 found Donna pleasantly plump, very pregnant, and running hard to catch Anna, who was rapidly becoming a two year old with the newfound power of vocabulary. She was working on some rudimentary verbal skills, like "mine" and "Dad, get that for me" and "No!" And Richmond was off stacking rocks somewhere. Think of that, setting stones for five months. Gee, sounds like fun, where do we sign up?

May 23, Kyle McFarren Breen arrived with a big smile on his face and hasn't stopped smiling since, which is somewhat amazing, considering the circumstances. In mid-August Kyle became ill with flu-like symptoms, and quit urinating. After a series of inconclusive tests at a Reno hospital, we took him to Children's Hospital at Stanford, approximately a five hours' drive. The doctors at Children's found a malignant cancerous tumor called neuroblastoma. It was the size of a baseball, located in his pelvis, near his bladder. Surgery was not an option, so the doctors started him on a chemotherapy program that has been on going since September. Kyle has had a great response to the chemo, and his tumor has shrunk approximately 50 percent already. He is doing so well the doctors feel he may be finished with the chemotherapy and CURED within a couple of months! The marvel of modern technology is truly amazing. Ten years ago there was no cure for this type of cancer. Kyle's cancer has been very challenging for us, but in some respects, a good experience. We have learned so much about health care, and we have had so much support from both our families and friends that much of this experience has been very positive. That's not to say this hasn't been very difficult because it has. Donna and Kyle are away from home a few days almost every week, at times as much as five to nine days in a row down at Stanford. Even though these HAVE been some hard days, we still feel very lucky because he has a cancer that can be cured, and to meet Kyle, you would never even know he was sick. He is so happy, bright and full of life.

I don't think we ever realized how much love and fear and tears our hearts could feel until now. I know we've aged a great deal the past few months, but somehow it feels okay...

I think you should stir the fire a bit, maybe even toss on another log, and we'll tell you a little more on a cheerier note.

You'd get a kick out of Anna Adair Breen. Way cute, plenty of curly blond locks, independence, sweetness and animation. Now where could she possibly have come by these traits? Recently she informed us that she was a pediatrician, helicopter pilot, who likes to take Stony Pony (our horse) for walks. Her evening prayer before dinner and/or bed, "Dear God, please help Kyle get better, Amen." She really cracks the whip on Dad, though. On the semi-daily runs through the park, if Dad doesn't push the stroller at the required pace, the command, "Faster, Farm boy, Faster" can be heard through the territory!

Meanwhile, Mom's home creating another culinary delight. Donna's skills in preparing wild game and vegetables are rapidly gaining world acclaim! Ah, yes, sun dried tomatoes, fresh herbs and garlic from the garden over a bed of pasta with a venison roast in a top secret super special sauce, followed by fresh apple pie! Hungry? Come on over for dinner. Give us a call! Donna is also in the running for Honorary RN of the Year, as well as Chauffeur Extraodinaire. She could probably drive to Stanford in her sleep and may have, once or twice. Her knowledge of Kyle's hematological, pharmaceutical and overall physiological condition is truly impressive.

Richmond and Tigger have been doing a somewhat commendable job of hunting and golfing (Tiggy is really good in the roughs and sand traps), planting trees, playing in the dirt, restoring historic buildings, wrestling railroad ties, stacking more rocks (at least a couple more months' worth), fishing, running, and wondering. Is this any way to run a business? I think I'll appoint Tigger CEO and take a vacation! I've got a better idea, let's all take a vacation. You can feel it, taste it, see it. You deserve it! White sand beaches, light tropical breezes, palm trees, warm blue waters, fresh fruit and fish, a tropical drink. Put that fire out. Let's Go!

We'll see you there. We love and miss you. Thanks for all your prayers. Merry Christmas and God Bless You!

We were leaving the hospital to go home on Christmas Eve. It was about 10 a.m.. Richmond and Anna had come down with Kyle and me; no matter what, we were going to be together on Christmas. The hospital often had a way of changing our plans. One day could lead to two, three, four or more. And the mountain pass could close with snow. With these considerations in mind, team traveling was the only way to go.

As we were leaving Children's Hospital that morning, a tall young man, about 18, was getting out of a car with his girlfriend and his mother. He had a Santa hat on his bald head, and a big bag of wrapped toys. He had the most beautiful smile and eyes. He looked at Anna, reached into his bag and gave her a little present. I almost burst into tears. He said he was going to the hospital because he just wanted to make sure none of the children were forgotten. It was a beautiful moment.

We arrived home at 7 p.m. We lit the Christmas lights on our small potted tree. The twinkling lights brought warmth to the room and spirit to the moment as we realized the thought of being in the hospital on Christmas was no longer a concern. It was also a great relief to be done with Round 4 of chemo. It hadn't gone very smoothly. Kyle continually threw up. There was great relief and joy gathered from being with each other. We were all very exhausted.

It was a wonderful Christmas. Next we had to watch his counts and see if we would escape F&N. After enjoying a few days at home, once again we were off to the hospital.

It seemed as though every holiday was marked by chemo, fever and neutropenia (F&N) or some other lovely test for poor Kyle. Missing out on New Year's Eve was no big deal. Richmond and I never went out on that night anyway, because there were too many lunatics driving drunk. Amateur Night. It was nice to arrive at Children's no later than dinnertime.

Upon arrival, I went and looked on the patient board, as usual. Cassie Lupro was in the hospital, so I went to see her and say, "Hi." It was Bob's birthday; so after the kids were in bed, we walked over to Pedro's for a cocktail.

It was nice to connect with friends who were in a similar situation. As different as all the cancers were, we still had a common thread to keep us together. We were all in the Chemo Club. We could laugh and tell really disgusting jokes that no one else would even utter out loud. Throwing up became known as, "the Technicolor Yawn."

The bartenders at Pedro's thought we were crazy, could barely believe that our kids all had cancer, and that was why we were all there. One night when there were four or five of us at Pedro's, one of the bartenders inquired, "Do you all work at Children's or do any of you have kids over there?" We all chuckled and replied, one-by-one, "My kid has cancer." The bartender was stunned.

Staying up to ring in the New Year was out of the question. I didn't want to celebrate badly enough to be tired and hung over the next day in a children's cancer ward. It would be no fun hearing people throwing up and feeling like doing it myself. So, New Year's Eve or not, Bob's birthday or not, back to Children's Hospital we went. We had loosened up a little bit and as far as I could tell, that was good therapy.

CHAPTER 5

LET THE FILMING BEGIN

Happy New Year!!

The family library was my first stop to check on the status of the camcorder. It was in—score! I was so excited to get to work on my film. Kyle seemed to be in good spirits even though he was sick all night. He had an IV in his head with a little mesh cap over it to keep it in place. We were going to unplug it, let it run on the battery, and cruise the hospital.

I put Kyle in his stroller and hooked the IV pole to the back. We were just about ready. But before going on our filming adventure, Kyle needed an appropriate party hat. On the front of his forehead, where the mesh cap was, I added a sign that said, "Happy New Year," and on the top I tied multicolored strands of curled ribbon. He was quite the party boy!

We started the film in our room. Kyle cooed and gurgled on cue. Our roommates were introduced and then we were on our way. First we went down and introduced Dr. Mark Mogul—The World Famous Oncologist. We asked him many embarrassing questions, including about his weight-loss program. He called it the "Humiliation Diet," as he would weigh himself in front of the nurses each Monday morning to check his progress, or lack thereof! He informed us that the Monday morning weigh-ins were on hold for a few weeks due to his holiday indulgence. (Mark could have stood to drop 10 pounds, but he was far from fat.)

After embarrassing Mark on film, he thought turnabout would be fair play. So he put Kyle and me on film. Dr. Mogul could have been a comedian, which is a fabulous talent to have in oncology.

A nurse named Cyd came by. She used to call Kyle, "Buck Shot."
"Did they have to shave Buck Shot's head for the IV?" she asked.
Some kids still had some hair, but I thought she was absolutely hysterical.
"No, silly," I said as I burst out laughing. "He was bald."
The next day: more transfusions—no big deal. I had faith in the blood being clean and there wasn't a choice, so on with the show. It was an everyday event: bags of blood going here, bags of platelets going there. Kids were walking around all the time with IV poles loaded with bags of this or that and more than one pump to make it all go. Joyce and Bob Lupro put goldfish in a bag for Cassie to have something fun to look at on her IV pole. Creativity was a tremendous asset that helped pass the hours.
The filming of the movie, "Hotel Auxiliary"—Auxiliary was the name of the cancer ward—continued. "Where the room service was awful, but the nurses were great."
Using the camera was a great diversion. The movie would serve its own purpose, allowing people to visualize where we were and what we did. I was planning on mailing copies of the tape to family members so they could see that we were doing OK.
The people in the lab couldn't believe I was filming everything. When I asked about the slides and cell counts, they took the time to explain what was what. At one point, a young woman asked if I wanted to see a slide with a bunch of white blood cells.
"Heck no!" I said, "I want to see Kyle's slide."
"His slide only has one white blood cell on it," she answered.
"That's OK," I said with a laugh. "I think it would be neat to see his."
She retrieved Kyle's slide and put it under the microscope. After looking through with my own eyes, I put the lens of the camcorder up to where an eye would rest. It was incredible to view and film his one white blood cell on that slide. We were all stunned that the camcorder had such focusing capabilities. The view was crystal clear. There, all by itself, was a circular cell, with another circle inside it. Not only were we passing the hours, but the information I was learning was interesting.

1/5/91 Personal

We have met some nice new people. Thomas is a real nice kid about 13. Yesterday was day #5 and it tends to be a break-down day. It was. A code blue also sounded at 4 p.m. on Babcock unit. The kid died. I didn't know her, but I was afraid it was Alena's boy. Alena bought Kyle a stuffed train with a music box in it. It was so thoughtful. Thomas can't breath very well and that makes me nervous along with the fact that he throws up often.

Today should be a better day, I told myself. I needed to spend more time taking care of myself, running or just getting out of the hospital. I went therapy-shopping and bought a sweater and shirt. It did some good. Alena seemed stressed and wanted to go over to Pedro's for a short one. The day had put me in touch with real-ity and the death issue. Talking with the nurses, they said that if a kid is that sick, they usually move him or her to a single room, because the other parents and kids don't need the extra stress. That was a relief, because I was worried that someone was going to die while I was eating my dinner or something.

The stress of hearing and seeing kids get sick all the time was often unnerving and patient confidentiality was greatly respected. There were times I said to myself, "If I hear that kid puke one more time, I'm going to puke!" Unless I knew the child or his or her parents well enough to have the inside story, I had no idea what to expect.

One night at Pedro's, with about five parents present, we decid-ed that hot dogs provided the best "Technicolor Yawn," because they looked exactly the same when some kid threw them up right back onto the plate. I think a few of Pedro's patrons moved out of earshot that night, which we also found quite amusing.

After too many days in a row at Children's Hospital, it was a good thing I had use of the camera. It was time to take it to Pedro's and film part of "Parent Therapy." It was quite the event! We all had an extra drink or two so we looked especially loose. The manager, Joe, already knew us and what our stories were. He always had a smile and kind word for us. At the end of the evening he took the camcorder so he could film us.

"Welcome to the Lifestyles of the Drunk and Disorderly," he narrated, mimicking Robin Leach. "These people are worth five-point-two billion dollars and no one knows why."

That was one of the more entertaining segments of our film.

I interviewed a wide assortment of people for my film. Nurses and doctors—even the man named Conrado at the cash register in the cafeteria. Every morning when I would get a tray to take out my breakfast, he would have a kind word and make me smile.

IT WAS DAY EIGHT OF our most recent stay. What's a girl to do when she's in need of a new 'do? Don't complain out loud in a cancer ward—most of the people there don't even have hair!

Even on my bad hair days, Kyle continued to keep a happy-go-lucky attitude. It was amazing considering all he had gone through. His blood counts were so low, he must have felt terrible. Day after day with Kyle having no neutrophils was unsettling.

The next day, we started a sequel to the movie, "Hotel Auxiliary," with Richmond, Anna and a cast of thousands. Richmond and Anna left, and Kyle and I prepared for a "field trip." After the nurse unhooked Kyle's IV, we went for a walk up to Palo Alto to have an ice cream or coffee.

By Day Twelve, our visit was growing old. I heard people say they had been at the hospital for 28 days for F&N. I hoped to God we wouldn't, but counted our blessings.

There were many areas of the hospital where Kyle and I ran into people. One was the women's room on auxiliary. It was a huge room with toilets on one side, a shower, then a tub and row of sinks. The toilets and shower/tub areas had curtains for privacy. It was there I met Monica Benninghoff, and she had been crying— a lot. She and her husband had just been told there was nothing else they could do for Chris. Monica and David were in their late thirties. They were kind, gracious and unassuming. They adored their children and though we had just met, we talked in depth. Chris had a sister named Jennifer, who at 10 was a lovely young girl with flowing blond hair. I could hardly conceive of what I had been told. It seemed so unacceptable. That was *that*? No alternative? Monica said they had told Chris about his counts and at age 8, he knew what they meant. I couldn't fathom it myself, yet an 8-year-old had the whole picture.

Our culture is totally inept at dealing with death. As if nobody ever really dies in America—except by accident. No one ever talks about it, yet each and every one of us will die. We're so unprepared. I've met so many people who've said, "Oh, he'll (Kyle) be OK." As if they thought if they kept saying it, it would become true. And we hoped it would be, but we knew then that we would be very lucky if Kyle survived.

JAN. 12, KYLE AND I finally were home. Hallelujah!

At a certain level, life had continued to go on without us. It was so strange to go home where Anna was doing everything a 2 1/2 year-old did. Richmond's business was busy as ever, and now we didn't have to listen to IV poles that never ceased beeping, because meds needed to be added or the cycles were complete. Kyle and I would sleep in our own beds—no nurses in and out of the room all night. I could snuggle with my husband, and boy did that feel good.

These times were incredibly difficult for Anna. She never knew if her mom would be there when she woke up and if mom was gone, she had no idea when she would be back. The daily phone calls when Kyle and I were gone were a double-edged sword. Anna needed to hear my voice, but it often left her in tears. Anna and I had big adjustments each time I was gone for awhile. She would rake me over the coals for two or three days, being especially difficult and demanding, then it was back to normal. Anna wasn't going to let me just walk in there and be her boss again, not without really working for it. It was a challenging few days, with my fatigue from all the hospital time an additional strain.

Noticing that pattern helped me come home and deal with being tortured by our toddler. She must have been very angry, though she never took it out on Kyle. It surprised me that she was so loving toward her brother. Anna would look at books with Kyle, get his stuffed animals and play games intermixed with lots of extra affection. She knew his cancer was why we were always gone—often on the spur of the moment.

Anna was very sharp. She had picked up on my eyelid test to see how low Kyle's hemoglobin was. Pulling gently on Kyle's lower lid revealed the wet area where one might fish out a piece of dirt causing irritation. If this area was very pale at the moment the lid was pulled down, his hemoglobin was usually very low. If the lid was quite red his hemoglobin count was usually fine. She would go up to Kyle and pull his eyelids down.

"Mom, I think Kyle is kind of pale," she'd say. "Should we go for a blood draw?"

A very unusual conversation to have with a 2 1/2 -year-old!

I was doing my prep work for dinner one afternoon when Anna came to me carrying her dolly and informed me, "My dolly's sick, so I'm taking her to the hospital."

"Great," I said. "I hope she gets better." I continued to work, thinking her comment was rather interesting.

A few minutes later she came back with her dolly.

"She's all better, Mommy!"

"Terrific," I said. "What did you do for her?"

"I gave her Cytoxan."

After I picked my face up off the floor, I casually replied, "That's great honey, as long as it makes her better."

I was flabbergasted. Not only was she playing let's-pretend with chemo, but she had even gotten the drug name correct. She blew my mind. At her age, I hadn't expected that, but then again, we hadn't expected cancer in the first place.

Richmond and I had always told Anna what was going on, what tests Kyle was having and what they were for. We had always believed that the more information she was given, the better off she'd be. We never told her that we were certain Kyle could conquer neuroblastoma; we told her that Richmond, I and she could try our very best to help him, and part of it was up to his little body. We were very positive thinkers, but we refused to tell her that we knew he would get better, because we simply didn't know for sure.

Anna almost always went along for Kyle's blood draws at Saint Mary's. She wanted to go to help Kyle and was terrific on many occasions. After the lab assistant had poked Kyle, she reassured him that he was OK and they were done.

It was so sweet to see her compassion for her brother. Usually a few kisses and hugs from her was all it took to get the smile back on his face. It was wonderful for her to be such a big help. She knew that she was helping him feel better.

CHAPTER 6

TESTS AND MORE TESTS

A series of tests would let the doctors know if Kyle's chemotherapy was working. The CAT scan, urine test and blood work weren't very difficult on him. But the bone aspiration was ugly.

After Kyle was sedated, Dr. Mogul stuck a tubular-shaped needle into him aiming for the pelvic bone. A screwing motion was used to extract a small piece of bone for the lab to evaluate. The test was very similar to the bone marrow aspiration, but more painful. It also filled me with anxiety. If the cancer had moved to Kyle's bones, the cancer prognosis would be much worse.

While he was under sedation, a bone scan was also done. Kyle was laid on a table where a long series of pictures were taken. That part didn't bother me. A number of hours before the test, I had to take Kyle to the same department for an injection that would help the doctors read the bone scan. The injection was radioactive, and was kept in a lead sheath so that the technologist wouldn't come in contact with this poisonous material. If that weren't bad enough, I was told, "Wash your hands thoroughly after every diaper change for 24 hours." I felt squeamish as I held Kyle and observed the tech administer the injection.

I stuffed a lot of that information so far back in my brain it was almost lost. If I thought about some of the things we did to Kyle in an effort to save his life or check on his progress, I would have self-destructed. Each time radioactive dye was pumped into his veins, or X-rays were taken or chemo was administered, I would chat with the administrative tech while mentally tuning out. It was a good thing that I was the "hospital parent" because

Richmond—a.k.a. Nature Boy—would have had a much more difficult time with some of the drug tests. He was a man who preferred all natural foods and spring water.

The constant blood draws and pokes for various reasons became a problem for me—not to mention Kyle. I used to help hold him while a nurse would start an IV or a phlebotomist would draw blood. Instead of them having to find another person to help, I could feel useful and Kyle would be done that much sooner. For a long time this system seemed to work just fine, but as he got a little older he started looking at me as if he wanted to know, "Why are you hurting me, Mommy?" That was the end of my being helpful. They could find someone else. I retired. In my new role I would "save" him from whomever was poking him when he was done. Kyle had been poked approximately 500 times in six months. I used to call the phlebotomist that poked Kyle most often the "Mosquito Woman." She loved coming to see Kyle, but hated to do his blood draw. Any time a vein was hit on the first try, we were thrilled.

One day, while waiting for transport to take us to one of Kyle's tests, I was pushing him through the hallway at Children's. I was bored and he was sedated, asleep on an angle in his stroller with his head tilted toward the side. His hemoglobin was low that day, leaving him rather pale. As I pushed the stroller past an office, a few of the women inside looked out at Kyle. A moment later one of them, a nurse, came out and approached me.

"Gosh, is your baby OK?" she said, maintaining a casual tone.

"Oh yeah," I replied, "he's just sleeping on sedation."

"I'm a nurse. Would it be all right if I checked him out?" she asked, rather sheepishly.

I just grinned and said quietly, "Sure, he does kind of look like the 'D' word, doesn't he?"

The look on her face was priceless. She must have felt as though I had read her mind.

An odd laugh accompanied a quick check on his vitals. He was fine and she relayed the results to her boss who had insisted, "Go check that kid out, he looks *really* bad."

One weekend at the beginning of February, Kyle spiked a fever, with low blood counts. Standing over his crib, I took his temperature as he slept. With chemo babies, their temperatures have to be taken under their arms. The rectum is not a choice because the chemo is so hard on the gastro-tract. Internal bleeding is a serious risk because the tissue is so fragile. Kyle slept on while I monitored his condition. His temperature was 101.5.

I started to pack, all the while looking outside while it continued to snow. I called the road report to see if the pass over Donner Summit on Interstate 80 was open. If too much snow fell, there was no way to get over. The report said chains were required. Mom was still awake, waiting, knowing a fever ultimately meant a trip over the mountains to Stanford, snow or not. It was late at night and we discussed the risks of traveling in blizzard conditions over a winding 10,000-foot pass.

First, however, we drove to the local ER. We waited patiently while the med orders were processed. Going to the hospital in the middle of the night was commonplace at that point in our lives. During times when Kyle's counts started to drop, I would tell Anna each night in bed that Kyle and I might not be there in the morning. She understood and would reassure me. "Mom, It's OK. I'll be fine." It was terribly hard on our little girl, yet she tried to be brave and supportive.

Had the weather been better, we would have been gone to Stanford; but the oncologist on call recommended traveling at the first light of day. The snow might let up and we would be well rested. He said he would rather have us there in one piece, and in any event, the ceftriaxone antibiotic would hold Kyle for a few more hours.

At 4 a.m., I loaded all of the bags for Kyle, Anna, Mom and myself into the Suburban for the trek over the mountains. Kyle and I would stay at the hospital while Mom and Anna stayed at the Hyatt. I brought Anna along for this reason: the doctors anticipated a lengthy surgery in the near future to remove the shrunken tumor. It would require a full day blocked out for the operating room in case of complications. Anna and I would be apart for a few weeks at that point, and we needed some time together, so we all went on this trip.

Anna loved being at the Hyatt with her grandma. Though quite young, she was already a great fan of jumbo shrimp cocktail arriving via room service. Mom and Anna spent most of their time visiting at the hospital. Richmond took a day off from the out-of-town job he was on and came over from Los Gatos the next day so we could all enjoy a day together. We hoped the proximity of his job would allow us more time together, but the commute was draining after already difficult days.

We were all trying to make the best of a tough situation. Anna played in the pre-school and went for walks with me while Mom sat with Kyle. The days dragged for Anna. Two-and-a-half-year-olds are very active and it was almost impossible to keep her occupied. It was much more difficult for me having her there, but it was important for her to be with me and understand where I was and what Kyle was doing when we were away from home.

As it turned out, we were in for some good news. A CAT scan showed the tumor had shrunk. Three days later—Feb. 9—we were going home. It was time to regroup before the surgery.

All of the tests had looked good and, best of all, the tumor was now only grape-size. Prior to chemo, the tumor had been baseball-sized and intertwined with Kyle's intestines. I had met with the surgical team, Dr. Schocat and Dr. Hartman. Kim and Jim Stone—our physician friends in Palo Alto who had opened their home to us—had told us that they were fantastic. Dr. Hartman had a good sense of humor and was easy to talk to. Schocat would do the surgery. He also seemed very nice, though more rigid. We felt very good about him being Kyle's surgeon.

Kyle's tumor was down on his pelvic floor, inside the body cavity at the bottom of the abdominal area. There were risks as with any surgery, and Kyle's were especially related to all the nerves located near the tumor. Nerve damage was a possibility. The areas of concern were loss of continence (being able to control the bladder and bowels) and loss of erections. Those were biggies and only offset by the knowledge that we had the best surgical team on Kyle's side. The doctors explained that the surgery would run four to five hours, if there were no complications. They would make an incision across Kyle's abdomen, gently move over his intestines and extract the tumor. If they couldn't reach all of it, they would flip him over and make an incision up the crack of his rear end. Hopefully, they would only have to make one incision.

Kim asked me what they were going to do. After telling her, she replied with true surgical humor, "Oh, they're going to do the baby fillet."

Kim and I became very close, crying together on many occasions in "my room" at their house. Her humor also made me laugh, and lightened up an otherwise frightening subject.

The next day, I saw Dr. Hartman before we left to go back to Reno. "Did you have any questions or need anything clarified before you and your husband come back down for Kyle's surgery?" he asked.

I couldn't pass up my opportunity to share a bit of physician humor. "It was explained well," I said. "If you can reach it all from the front, great; if not, you'll flip him over and do the old baby fillet."

The look on Dr. Hartman's face was priceless.

Home we went. It was time to gather our wits and strength. Surgery was as serious as it got.

Mom had been with us for about a month, and though she would never say it, I'm sure we were driving her a little bit crazy. Not to mention that she had so generously put her life on hold. She was flying home to Dallas now, and Dawn, my sister, was flying into Palo Alto. Richmond, Anna and I would be going down for the surgery. As difficult as it would be, Kyle was her brother, and Anna deserved to be there, too.

The nress comes
and brings every-
thing he needs.

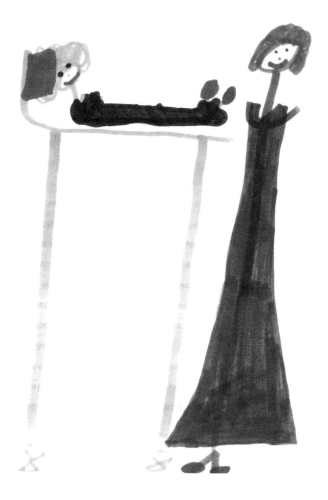

CHAPTER 7

MAJOR SURGERY

We arrived at Stanford Medical Center to check in for pre-op. Surgery, Intensive Care Unit (ICU) and regular pediatrics were there, and so the procedures would be performed at the medical center, not Children's Hospital.

Richmond, Anna and I slept at Kim and Jim's that night. At Peds (pediatrics) there wasn't anywhere to sleep, whereas at Children's most of the parents stayed bedside on rollaway cots. After talking to Dr. Schocat and Dr. Hartman, we decided to come to the hospital as soon as we were up and running, but we didn't intend to be there when Kyle was brought in to surgery. They were taking him at 6 a.m. for surgery at 6:45. There would only be about 10 minutes between waking him up and putting him under a general anesthetic. It wouldn't be possible to breast-feed Kyle for days after the operation. We had already been told that disturbing the intestines in any way during surgery would result in them shutting down for a period of about a week. Until then nothing could go in, since nothing would come out.

We arrived at the hospital about 9 a.m. and went up to the waiting area outside of the pediatric ICU. Dr. Schocat was going to look for us there as soon as surgery was complete. Dawn had flown in the night before so she could be with us for extra support. Dawn's husband, Mike, was a terrific guy who loved to tease; but when it came to family matters such as Kyle's, he was behind Dawn completely and would do anything to help. Dawn and Mike had raised their two daughters, Kelly and Erin, the same way. Family came first.

The stress was so high with so much riding on this surgery. We all had our coping mechanisms. One of Richmond's was to go for a long run. When he asked me if I minded if he went running, I just smiled and told him to run as long as he needed to. Kyle wasn't due out of surgery for hours, and I was used to endless waiting at the hospital.

Dr. Schocat was going to be able to do a preliminary biopsy on the remaining tumor. It wouldn't be conclusive but would give us more information. One of the possible characteristics of neuroblastoma after chemo is that it can mature into a benign form called ganglioneuroma. That would be great and was one of our hopes.

Richmond returned from his much-needed run. After about 10 miles his stress level had dropped quite a bit. He told me that during his run a wonderful thing had happened. All through the week prior to surgery he had been in a very sad, depressed and frightened state of mind. Basically, he was scared by death, as we all were. He had no positive energy at all and felt very bad that he was unable to muster up any strength and "positive vibes" to put out for Kyle. When he left for his run he didn't know if he could even go a quarter-mile.

As his run progressed, he found himself flooded with energy and emotion. His pace became meteoric. Suddenly, an abundance of powerfully positive energy was flowing through him. He began to cry as he ran near the hospital grounds and knew this energy was meant for Kyle and the doctors and nurses who were operating on him. Concentrating and focusing this energy toward Kyle and the doctors, Richmond finished his run at a lightning pace with a wonderful feeling of renewed energy and hope.

KYLE WAS OUT OF surgery at 11:45 a.m. We all stood up when Dr. Schocat walked into the waiting area. He said everything had gone well and Kyle had responded like a trooper. Dr. Schocat said he had removed all he could see or feel of an encapsulated tumor: one that is harder on the outside and softer on the inside. It was very small—the size of a grape—and looked alive in the middle. He cut it open in surgery. Kyle would be in ICU as soon as the recovery staff sent him up. We could see him when he arrived.

A short time later, an ICU nurse said we could see Kyle. He was asleep and wired for sound. There were so many tubes and monitors attached to our little baby's body that our hearts felt heavy. We were very hospital savvy by now, but this sight was one more reminder that this was extremely serious business. There wasn't much to say to each other, so Richmond, Dawn and I just took turns standing by his bed. When Kyle woke up, Richmond and I told him how much we loved him, stroked his bald little head and gave him kisses. The little baby that never quit smiling looked up at us with weary eyes. We brought Anna to his bedside and she looked down at him compassionately.

"Hi Kyle, I love you."

He looked up at her and smiled. That really drove home how important the entire family unit was. She was only allowed in ICU for a few minutes at a time, yet she had accomplished what we could not. I was so glad we had decided to bring her down for such a big surgery.

Each ensuing day we spent much of our time at the hospital. Kyle was still "totally tubular," so we weren't able to pick him up, and his intestines still weren't functioning so he couldn't eat. He was fed via IV. Richmond, Dawn and I took turns sitting bedside. Kyle had been moved to the pediatric unit know as "Peds B" and was progressing well. He slept quite a bit, and during these times we would go for walks. It was wonderful having Stanford Mall next to the hospital. It's a very high-end shopping center with lots of great places to eat. We sat at an outdoor cafe for lunch with a glass of wine to take the edge off. It was nice to feel the sunshine and smell the fresh air after feeling so cooped up at the hospital.

Richmond and Anna were going to return to Reno in the morning. The rest of Kyle's hospital time was waiting—the critical part was over. That afternoon, Dr. Schocat found Richmond and me and gave us the update on Kyle's condition. The final on pathology proclaimed Kyle cancer-free!!

Down came the flood gates, out poured tears of joy. We had been so afraid the tumor contained live cells and we would have to put Kyle through more chemo. Our relief was unbelievable. As I stood there hugging Richmond and then Dr. Schocat, I felt like we had just been given our lives back. We no longer belonged to cancer.

RICHMOND CAME AND SAID good-bye to Kyle and let him know he would see him in a few days. He and Anna had been in Palo Alto for five days. They would return to Reno, and Dawn would stay through the week to keep me company. Dawn and I always had a blast together. We loved sick humor and had gained plenty of material to work with at the hospital. Dawn and I had a couple of days together before she had to fly back to Chicago to be with her husband and kids. We stayed at Kim and Jim's and enjoyed dining out each night. Richmond thought we deserved it and encouraged us to go to some good restaurants and enjoy our time together. Even Dawn, who could tease unmercifully, had to admit Richmond was terrific.

Three days later, Kyle was ready for his first day of fluids. Yet I had come down with a terrible cold.

Feeling too sick to get out of bed after having waited what felt like forever to breast-feed Kyle, I not only felt awful, but was guilt-ridden that my baby would feel abandoned. My tears flowed. He didn't seem too upset by it all as far as the nurses could tell. Kyle drank his formula from a bottle and was probably so tickled someone gave him fluids, he didn't care who it was. We never brought anything to eat or drink into the room. The following day was his first bite of food in nine days. He was pretty pleased and soon we would be able to go home. The whole idea of just leaving was bizarre. We had spent so much time at the hospital and met so many wonderful people, it seemed almost like home.

Two days later, the last tube—the Hickman—was removed from Kyle's little body. His temperature returned to normal.

We would be leaving in the morning. The Hickman that was removed would have served as a permanent IV access had the operation shown a need for more chemo. A Hickman is a plastic tube that enters at the middle of the chest and goes under the skin toward the neck, down a big vein that ends up at the heart. Kids who continued with chemo didn't get pokes if they had a Hickman. A wave of relief swept over me as I realized removal of the Hickman also meant I wouldn't need to learn to care for a Hickman.

Odd as it seemed, our imminent departure brought mixed emotions. My journal entries explain:

2/21/91 Personal
*Today is bittersweet. A little girl named Janet died last night.
Thank God and rest her soul. I talked to her mom the other
day and saw her condition—which was scary—to say the
least. I will write her parents. I don't know what I'll say...
More bad news. Cassie Lupro is out of remission. Joyce, Tyson
and Nicole flew from Alaska to be with Cassie and Bob. I put
in a call to their San Jose number and talked to Joyce's mom.
I'll try again later. RHB and I went to CH@S before he left to
thank numerous people. Very emotional for both of us. We'll
miss lots of people that were so good to us that I don't know
if I (we) could of made it without them.*

*I called the Lupros tonight. Bob said Cassie got hit with the
big big guns last night, and was very sick, though doing fairly well this morning. I pray for her remission.*

*The cancer world is so cruel. We can't have a clean, clear,
happy victory. Even cancer won't allow that unless you are
completely heartless and uncaring. We are getting ready to go
home and celebrate life, but we leave knowing Janet has just
died, a kid on the next ward right behind her and Cassie our
dear friend is out of remission. This is what the cancer world
is like. There will never be a united victory, just singular cures
and remissions in the big war. That doesn't make our victory
any less real, just less exciting and a cancer reality is
attached saying, "Not everyone is that lucky."*

We don't forget.

*We are so thankful and almost embarrassed to tell some of
our less fortunate friends down here. They are all happy for
us, and we all need to know, "There have got to be some winners." (Monica Benninghoff.) This keeps all of us going. But I
feel so bad knowing so many of my friends' kids are dying.*

*We are now a part of the outside world because we are cancer-
less. We will try to fit into the "real" world again. I know we can,
but a certain fear is attached. It feels like forever since I've lived
"there." I'll hardly know how to act. We'll adjust. But Kansas
won't be the same anymore. That much we know for sure.*

*There has almost been a fear since Kyle has been cancer-free, but
that fear is starting to lift and I'm starting to get excited about
going home. I know I'll (we'll) still visit all our old friends.*

*I have always had a hard time leaving a place that was good
to me.*

*CH@S was good to us. They gave us Kyle's life back. There
could never be a better gift. This will be the close of a very special chapter in our lives.*

Kyle had a fever Feb. 22, forcing us to stay an extra day. Then we were off for good.

I kept thinking about how lucky we were. We were "cured"— that was it. I felt awful for all those poor people in remission. It seemed like they were walking around with an ax tied by a string hanging edge-down over their heads, and every day a guy walked through town with this huge pair of shears that could cut the string holding the ax. No one ever knew if it was his day. I felt so bad for all those people. Every day mattered. Don't sweat the small stuff. We had many friends in the Land of Uncertainty and visits to make before we went back to Reno.

Kyle and I went over to Children's (we had been in Stanford) and visited with nurses, doctors and friends. I wanted to thank everyone I could for everything they had done for us. Friends were the sanity life-line for me. Kyle's life-line was more literal: I wanted all the doctors and nurses to know how important they were to us and how much they had helped make our lives pleasant under extremely trying conditions.

Finally, Kyle and I buckled up in our truck, and pulled out of Children's parking lot.

"Good-bye Children's," I cried out, sobbing. "I love you."

CHAPTER 8

H O M E   A T   L A S T

So there we were. Home, together, and with the best news we could have possibly imagined.

"Hey buddy…why is your wife crying so much?"

"Oh I don't know…our son was just pronounced cancer-free and she didn't want to leave the cancer ward."

Strange as it sounded, my heart was heavy and I cried for five days feeling as though I had a popsicle on a 100-degree day and my friends were lying in the hot sand. Walking away felt like betrayal.

We did a lot of talking that week. After talking with the Lupros one day I approached Richmond.

"Maybe I should drive down to "Chaz" (my abbreviation for Children's Hospital at Stanford) to see them."

He knew his wife wasn't mentally all back yet, and calmly replied, "Donna, you're not going to Stanford. You're staying here. We need you."

He was right, but I also felt like a deserter who had gotten a lifeboat, hopped in and left everybody else on a sinking ship. I almost felt guilty that Kyle had survived when so many had died before him and would continue to die after him. Monica Benninghoff, another cancer mom, had said, "There have got to be some winners," and I needed to remember that.

It felt strange being home, knowing we wouldn't have to go back except for checkups. We were no longer active members of the Chemo Club.

Being on the outside was so weird. The only places I'd spent time when Kyle was sick were the grocery store, home and the hospital. We were all going to need to do some serious regrouping. Anna wasn't sure who was the boss. After all, I had been gone a lot and she was doing pretty well without me. Richmond was happy to turn over the boss duties since I had always been the heavy and he had the role of softy.

Our regrouping went one day at a time. It meant waking up with the conscious realization that we didn't have to go to the hospital for any reason. No blood draws, no transfusions, nothing. Kyle had received approximately 24 transfusions. We kept faith that all the transfusion blood was "clean." Cancer had been enough; we didn't want to have to deal with AIDS, too.

Each day, another pebble fell to the ground off our shoulders. There was still a truck-load left, but we were starting to feel better. We tried to relax and let normal life flow out of what had been an incredibly bizarre experience.

I kept in contact with most of my hospital friends via frequent phone calls. Kendra was in the middle of what would be a long protocol of chemo for her rhabdomyosarcoma. It was a tumor that she had discovered on her thigh. Her chemo was going well and she continually amazed me with her humor and courage.

One of the drugs they gave her had a side-effect called "drop foot." That is what happens when someone walks and instead of the heel of the foot touching first, the toes drop as if the muscles don't exist. At that point Kendra had a walker to help her stay mobile. Normally, she would have been screaming down a mountain on skis this time of the year. The walker was a complete change of pace for her.

I had stopped by her hospital room one afternoon before Kyle and I left. She was talking to her doctor. I didn't know what her request was, but she was demanding something in her usual humorous style.

"Dr. Louie," she said, "You better listen to me or I'll have to put my drop-foot down."

He smiled, enjoying her incredible humor.

Kendra never saw the bad, only the good. Her parents, Sharon and David, are wonderful people who always had something pleasant to say or words of encouragement. We had many chats, exchanging medical information and other anecdotes. I could see where Kendra's zest for life came from.

I tried to keep my question of "why?" to a minimum. But on occasion I couldn't help but ask myself, "Why do the nice people get cancer and the world is full of bad guys who seem to remain healthy?" I just didn't understand. Of course, there are no answers to those kinds of questions. We had to make the best of it instead of expending energy decrying life's incongruities.

The comfort of family and home felt wonderful. I loved to cook and was enjoying the luxury of having a full spice cabinet and a freezer that held lots of delectable choices. It beat cooking in the patients' lounge.

Every day I would catch myself mentally drifting back to the hospital. I had missed being in my own bed at night. As nice as it was being able to sleep bedside when Kyle was in-patient, finding a good cot was always a challenge. Not only was comfort an issue, but each morning by 8 a.m. beds were to be folded up and moved off to the side. Being at home where I could wander up to my room any old time and lie on my own bed was great! Having a wonderful husband to lie next to every night was even better.

I hardly knew what to do with my time, now that we could lead normal lives. Let's see…there was laundry, cooking and cleaning and, wow—there was a lot of free time with the hospital out of the picture. Anna, Kyle and I spent hours lying on the carpet in the afternoon sun, reading and laughing. We went to the park and ran around. It all seemed so incredibly simple and perfect. How could people complain about some of the insignificant things that upset them so much? It just didn't make sense anymore. We had a whole new looking glass in which we viewed a completely different world. And this world was a wonderful one.

Richmond enjoyed having his wife back. It took me weeks to grasp the idea that our bags didn't have to be packed anymore. We could actually make social plans with no concerns regarding low blood counts or that Kyle might need a transfusion.

As days continued to pass, I was feeling more and more comfortable on the outside. On the inside, I was still mortified and worried constantly about our friends who were still back at Children's. The best therapy was living for the moment and enjoying my family. Kyle and Anna played so wonderfully together that it often brought tears to my eyes. They were so darn cute and

Anna was so protective. Watching them play with Richmond was a true joy.

I spent time pouring over my cooking magazines, getting delightful recipes to tantalize my family's taste buds. Anna was quite the little gourmet, and enjoyed the most unusual dishes. Sushi, curried chicken or venison with juniper berries would all be terrific choices for her. We were adjusting and doing things we did before Kyle was diagnosed, but we knew in our hearts that life would never be the same. And that was fine, because there were things that would be better. I have met people who almost seemed burdened by their children. There would not be a single day that we wouldn't thank God for ours.

ONE MORNING, I CALLED Monica to check on Chris, knowing his body wouldn't be able to hold out much longer. She said he was still hanging on, but just barely. We chatted for a few minutes and I let her know I would call again soon. A few days later, I woke up as usual around 6:30 a.m. I was still in a dream when I started to awaken. In the dream I was at Children's Hospital. I wasn't really in the dream; I was more like an observer. The room radiated a very, very white light and doctors and nurses were all standing around what I knew was Chris' bed. It was very peaceful with a tranquillity that engulfed the room. I woke up thinking, "Wow, that was weird. I think I'll check on Chris this morning."

About an hour later, after Richmond left for work, I called Children's and asked if Chris Benninghoff was in-patient. They transferred me to his room. After a few rings, Monica answered.

"Hello."

"Monica? This doesn't sound like you. If this is a bad time, I can call back," I said.

"No...it's O.K...." She replied. "But Chris just died about a half an hour ago."

We only talked for a few more minutes and I was stunned at how calm she seemed. I'm sure she was in shock. The finality of death is so overwhelming. (It wasn't until months later that I told her about my dream. Chris had indeed died in a setting resembling my dream.) As I hung up, I was overcome with a flood of emotions knowing it was a blessing that Chris was no longer in pain; but it was all so awful that it also filled me with anger. They were wonderful people. How could this happen? I had said enough prayers to sink a battleship. And this was the result? Was anyone up there listening?!

On a day like that I wondered and felt especially afraid. Having no control was awful. Being unable to help a friend felt even worse. That day, I was devastated. Tears clouded my every thought. Tears of fear, compassion, anger and sadness. Fear of losing more friends, compassion for the pain and suffering already passed, and anger that covered a multitude of subjects. I was angry at God. I was angry at people for being so petty. I felt like yelling at the person in the grocery line who complained because it took an extra two minutes. It was hard for me to see people worrying about "the small stuff." I was angry because everyone always said, "It will be OK." For the little things in life, that rule applied. When the larger issues were at hand it would be best if people said nothing.

It had only been 14 days since we had left Stanford. I was trying to recover and focus on the present, not live in fear of the unknown. Chris had a totally different disease than Kyle; and intellectually, I knew that was everything.

But emotionally, we were comrades and their loss was our loss.

I WAS STARTING TO FEEL a consuming desire to "give something back." I really didn't know what I could do, but I needed to make a contribution.

Kyle's first checkup was scheduled for the following week: an MRI (magnetic resonance image) to check out his insides, as well as blood and urine tests, were on the schedule.

I wasn't the least bit worried about the upcoming tests. We had dealt with the best doctors in the country and they felt Kyle was cancer-free. Who was I to argue? Richmond wasn't quite as confident, but still felt very optimistic.

Kyle and I drove down on March 24 for his morning appointment the next day. We would be back for Richmond's birthday on the 26th. Birthdays and other holidays weren't that important to us, but it was nice to keep them hospital-free.

3/24/91 Personal
Today I went back to CH@S for the first time post cancer. It felt good. The Lupro's were the only ones there that I knew of the families. Cassie is not in the best shape, though all things con-

sidered she's doing well. They are hoping for a good bone marrow match. But even with one, the chances aren't that good. The chances for Cassie's survival are very poor. Joyce seems to have a handle on it and has decided in her own mind that if Cassie's body can do it, she'll be all right, if not she'll die. They are very strong. Sometimes I feel like screaming at the rest of the world, 'Quit your bitching!' People complain about the most ridiculous things.

3/26/91 Personal
Happy Birthday Richmond. I am stuck at Kim and Jim's in Palo Alto due to snow on the mountain. It seems as if all the holidays have been marked with a visit to CH@S this last year. While I'd rather be at home today, the only thing that matters is Kyle's MRI was clear as a bell.

We don't have to be back for 2 months and this extra time to visit my friends at Children's is really nice. Thomas is still in, and looking worse for the wear. He has rhabdo (rhabdomyosarcoma), and isn't doing well. I'll go visit him today.

I am starting to feel like an outsider looking in—and it doesn't feel bad.

I saw the Lindemann's from Bend, Oregon again. Bad news. Pat is out of remission—again—less than 3 weeks later—it's very, very bad. I didn't see Pat. I should go see him in the hospital tomorrow before we leave. They'll (the doctors) probably be blasting him with major chemo ASAP.

Thomas looks trashed. I visited him today and told him I'd call him. He needs some extra support. He is an absolute mess. His mouth looks like an aliens.

These poor kids.

Tonight Bob, myself and a couple named Hal and Norma went to Pedro's for Therapy. We had a really nice time. They are all really good friends. I missed Alena and we did a shot of tequila for her. We had some really good talks and a real nice time.

I am a lucky lady.

I love you Richmond and Anna and miss you both a bunch.

The next morning, the snow cleared and the pass was open. Kyle and I drove in our trusty truck. Nothing could stop us now! We had a clear MRI and the world in our hands. With a clear scan our future looked better every day. I still felt this overwhelming desire to do some good for the cancer community. I started to consider orchestrating a bone marrow drive. Some of the kids we knew were in serious trouble and needed compatible bone-marrow donors for transplants.

A bone-marrow transplant, as I understood it, required a blast of chemo so big it pretty much killed the patient. At the last minute, the life-saving marrow from a healthy compatible donor was transfused into the cancer patient. The bone marrow found its way to the bones and started producing healthy blood cells, which in turn saved the patient's life. I never understood how the new bone marrow knew where to go because it was put into an IV, not stuck into the patient's bones. Science is amazing and the human body continued to astound me.

A transplant sounded feasible but…there was a catch. A donor is very difficult to find. Blood type is easy to match, but bone marrow requires six parts of the blood to match. What parts? I didn't know! A biological sibling's chance of matching are only 1 in 4. Once outside of that immediate circle, the odds increase to 1 in 20,000.

It was not like going down for a pint of B+ blood. Bone marrow matching is really complicated and confusing. Cassie was adopted by the Lupros and the birth mother had no other children by the same father. Bob and Joyce exhausted every possible avenue trying to find a donor.

Cassie needed a transplant or she was going to die. Bob and Joyce had been my best friends at the hospital and I couldn't just stand by without doing something!

CHAPTER 9

THE BONE MARROW REGISTRY DRIVE

A bone marrow drive would require a lot of work. I contacted Heart of America Bone Marrow Donor Registry for information on organizing a drive. I also contacted United Blood Services, explained what I wanted to do, and sought information and help to conduct a successful drive. After very little research, I realized the primary goals were fund-raising and education.

A person can be on the registry for years and never be contacted as someone's potential match. The test for the Bone Marrow Registry Drive requires one small vial of blood to be drawn. No bone marrow—just blood. That sample is mailed to one of the few labs in the country that can do the breakdown for compatibility. The cost of each test was $65. After the sample breakdown is complete, the information is entered into the national registry.

I knew the chance of finding a match for Cassie was slim, but I needed to do something and that was her only hope. If a match for anyone, anywhere, was found that would be terrific.

I started calling people in town for support. The drive required publicity and financial aid. My goal was 100 registry donors. I always believed that if I had a really good cause, people would help support it. But I learned that raising money was tough. My original expectations were far greater than the reality of two weeks of knocking on doors and talking with people on the phone.

The local Junior League gave me guidance. Members had a lot of experience with women's groups and raising money. We developed a flier, and our local grocer/drug center—Raleys—donated 50 copies of a picture I took of Bob, Cassie and Joyce. The fliers were printed and I attached the photos.

One evening after the children were in bed, Richmond was keeping me company while I finished the fliers. I borrowed a paper cutter to crop the photos to the size we needed. That meant leaving Bob out of the picture. I've always been a photo nut and knew what we needed to do the job. I worked quickly, cropping the photos to the finished product size. While working on the fliers, I sat there looking at 50 Bobs—and a light bulb went off in my mind. I went to our junk drawer and retrieved a half-dozen pairs of chopsticks. While splitting the chopsticks apart, I broke into uncontrollable laughter. Richmond had no idea what I was laughing about. I tried to catch my breath, sipped my wine and explained, "We'll make Bob stir sticks!" More laughter followed by more giggles. I glued Bobs back-to-back on each stir stick cut to match. "Hey—having a bad day? Don't want to drink alone? Stir one up with Bob!"

We must have laughed off and on for two hours that night. "Bob can dance," twirl, twirl went the Bob stir stick. Making my little art project kept the entertainment rolling. After all, Bob and I stirred one up at Pedro's on many occasions and that had been good therapy. By the end of the night there were about 10 Bob stir sticks in our kitchen, the fliers for the Bone Marrow Registry Drive were complete, and Richmond and I were both tired but felt good about what we were doing.

People wanted to know what it took to donate bone marrow if they were compatible donors. It was an in-patient procedure done under a general anesthetic. A large needle made 25 to 30 punctures into the pelvic bones and sucked out bone marrow. It literally sounded like a big pain in the rear end—but big deal! A few Tylenol pills for a few days and a donor would be back in the saddle. Someone else would have a whole new chance at life and the donor's bone marrow would rejuvenate itself. The patient would also pay for the procedure-related expenses of the donor.

I continued to meet with some people in the community. The power company had sponsored blood drives and officials were very interested, but couldn't fit into Cassie's time frame. (They did conduct a bone marrow registry drive, due in part to my efforts, at a later date and actually had a match within their company!)

A local real estate organization brought me to its weekly meeting. Standing up in front of a room of about 20 men and women, holding Kyle, I explained what we had already been through and the proposed effort to help others less fortunate. After asking each one of them to be a donor, or provide $65 for someone who was willing to be on the registry but didn't have the money, they generously contributed more than $1,200. In all, a total of $6,500 was raised—providing enough money for 100 donors to participate in the program.

During the fund-raising, a young television newscaster offered to do a spot on her station. Kyle and I met with her and recorded what ultimately was a terrific little spot on the 5 o'clock news. The word was getting around, and we were hoping for a good turnout.

Then the Lupros called with bad news. Cassie was at the stage where she was too sick for a transplant. The chances of her regaining remission were impossible, barring divine intervention. The sadness I felt for them engulfed me, leaving my heart so heavy I felt it sinking every time I thought of Cassie and her family. The drive would go on and hopefully someone somewhere would get a second chance at life. The bone marrow drive was scheduled for May 5, 1991. It was a great success. One hundred new people joining the bone marrow registry. I felt great about my accomplishment.

While I was busy with the drive, Richmond was busy working on a letter to let our friends and loved ones know about Kyle's good health. Richmond's family (the Breens) have lived in Nevada for many generations. There were a lot of local people who watched Richmond grow up and many were watching and wondering if Kyle would get to grow up. Anna was going to turn 3 the next month, and Kyle would reach his first birthday.

We both worked to finish the letter and got it mailed out. By the time we put the envelopes in a post office box, the date was a few weeks old, but that was OK.

"KYLE MCFARREN BREEN IS A HAPPY HEALTHY BOY!" the letter began.

"The impact of the last seven months upon our lives is as yet hard to comprehend," we wrote.

"It was as if we were standing in the middle of the Black Rock Desert on a warm, crystalline blue day when suddenly a fierce and powerful dust devil slammed into us, spun us, then threw us to the ground while blinding us with stinging alkali dust.

"And then it was gone. And it was a beautiful crystalline blue sky day once again..."

CHAPTER 10

BIRTHDAYS AND A CHECK-UP

I continued to keep in touch with our friends at Children's. Kyle's appointment was scheduled for May 20. Anna's birthday was May 18 and Kyle's five days later. We decided halfway through mailing the letters that we should include a flier for a party.

We didn't want to leave Anna out or do anything that would make her feel any less special. She had dealt with that plenty in the last year. We had a party just for her with some of her little friends on the 18th. I would be leaving with Kyle for Stanford the next day.

The flier invited about 250 people to celebrate life and birthdays with champagne and hors d'oeuvres. On the way down to Stanford I stopped in Napa Valley and bought cases of champagne. A good friend generously allowed us a grower's discount on all the cases, saving us a lot of money. She joked with me, asking if I didn't feel like I was jinxing Kyle's upcoming appointment. I said, "I don't think it's *really* possible…but if it is I hope I paid off the voodoo cancer gods with the bone marrow drive."

We laughed as I loaded the champagne in my truck and covered it to deter thieves.

Friends from far and wide were invited to our celebration of life. Many couldn't make it due to short notice, but quite a few were planning on partying at our place on May 25.

Kyle and I arrived at Children's for his checkup. First we went down to Day Hospital and Auxiliary to see if any of our friends were there. The Lupros were in. It was always wonderful to see them. Though we didn't get to see Tyson and Nicole often, we had grown to love the whole family. Bob and Cassie had stopped in Reno overnight on the way to a ski trip in Utah earlier that spring. Cassie still felt pretty good then, and enjoying life to its fullest was the order of business. Cassie and Anna jumped on the beds pretending they were kangaroos with their arms bent in front, giggling nonstop.

I told Bob and Joyce we were going to get an MRI, first thing, then I'd see them back at clinic. After sedation and Kyle's MRI, it was down to the lab for blood, up to the clinic for urine and then, finally, to the waiting area. After waiting awhile, the Lupros came in, pulled me aside and asked if I could keep Cassie for awhile because the doctors were giving them the "there's *nothing* else we can do" speech. They really didn't want Cassie to be there. "No problem," I said. "I'll either be in the clinic waiting area or in a room waiting to talk to Dr. Mogul about Kyle's results. You can bring Cassie to whichever room we're in." It was the least I could do for them on a day like that.

I still couldn't believe all the treatments were exhausted on Cassie's behalf. Denial made a serious play in my mind, trying to establish a good foothold. We were at one of the finest children's hospitals in the country, maybe the world. I met people that brought their child from as far as South Korea in hopes of curing that child's cancer. Keeping myself together for Cassie, Bob and Joyce would be necessary.

I was standing waiting at the clinic counter chatting with Marcia. She was the "busiest woman ever," running the clinic with nary an idle moment. She probably got tired of my bugging her, so she sent us to a room to wait. I was sitting there holding Kyle, talking to him about silly baby things, when in walked Dr. Mark Mogul, a.k.a. Mark, a.k.a. Dr. Mogulley—World Famous Oncologist. By this time in our relationship we had crossed the patient-doctor barrier into friendship, so I started chatting with him.

A funny look was on his face. Not Mark's standard funny face, but something a little more serious. I paused (once in awhile I knew when to be quiet) and waited for his comments.

Mark looked at me with gentle eyes and calmly said, "The MRI shows there's another tumor where the old one was."

"What?!" I shrieked. "No Way!"

At that instant I heard a knock. Joyce opened the door and let Cassie in. I looked up at Joyce.

"Kyle has a new tumor," I stated matter-of-factly. "Take all the time you need."

As it turned out she didn't hear me; so Cassie, who had sat through many of these conversations, just hung out with Kyle, Dr. Mark, and me.

Dr. Mark proceeded to tell me what the recommended treatments and timetable were for Kyle. He proposed four rounds of Group B chemo. Day 1 being cisplatin, Day 3 being VP-16, every 28 days. These were the big guns, with the possibility of serious side-effects. I was astonished. I just sat there in a fog thinking, how can this be? *Didn't we already do this?* Feeling like I was in The Twilight Zone, we calmly discussed the urgency of surgery for complete removal of the tumor followed by chemo and possibly radiation.

"Oh my God," I muttered. "Here we go again."

I felt my body begin to go numb as I slipped into mental shock.

Dr. Mark answered all of my questions and was the most supportive doctor and person I could have dealt with. We were incredibly blessed to have him for Kyle's doctor.

Cassie, Kyle and I walked down the hallway. As my feet fell one in front of the other, I felt as though they weren't attached to my body. I was bewildered. Kyle was his usual animated self and Cassie was content to be with us while her parents were busy. Cassie had heard that kind of conversation for much of her life— tumor here, lump there, chemo this, X-ray that. No new news there. We continued to wander down the hall.

Bob and Joyce came around a corner looking for us. Their talk had been awful, driving the denial further away.

"Did you hear what I said when you left Cassie in our clinic room?" I asked Joyce.

"No," she said, "I didn't really catch it."

"Kyle relapsed," I told Bob and Joyce. "There is a tumor about the size of the one they took out in the same place."

Their lives were slammed by another cruel blow from the beast cancer. We all hugged each other and went out to the back of the hospital. We grabbed a bedspread out of a linen closet on our way out to the lawn that bordered the rear entrance of the hospital. We laid out the bedspread on the grass and sat down. We were all stunned, except for the kids. Children have this wonderful superman/woman mentality. "It's OK! I'm invincible!" So much of it rolled right off their backs. Kyle was too young to know, but I saw it in older children. They never seemed to worry about dying.

We sat there for quite awhile talking about life's challenges, all the while wondering what our futures held. It was a blessing that we had each other to lean on; and it was especially important because both of our families were split up much of the time, due to the cancer war.

Joyce and Bob took turns being at Stanford in the winter. Bob drove a cement truck, and in Juneau there wasn't a lot of cement being poured in the winter months. Sometimes their whole family was at Stanford or in Juneau, depending on Cassie's medical schedule. Richmond and I were split up during medical gigs, but fortunately, Reno was closer to Palo Alto. Once again, I had gone to Stanford alone with our baby because I was sure I could handle the tests and I really didn't think there would be a problem. Once, maybe; twice—no way! Now I had to get on a phone and tell my husband, long-distance, that our son had relapsed.

Richmond knew immediately from my tone that there was trouble. I told him straight out what the tests had shown. The silence that ensued over the phone was paralyzing, while the rage and insanity in our minds was deafening. We were both too shocked to cry; the tears would come later.

Almost absurdly, there was another problem. Somewhere in the neighborhood of 200 people were going to show up at our home for a party in four days. Deborah, Richmond's sister, took the job of calling each and everyone to let them know the party was off. I don't know how she pulled it off, but only one couple showed up that day. (Seeing their expressions plummet into despair was a clear illustration of what was happening in our lives.)

Knowing three cases of champagne were in the front of my truck with no party to go to, Bob, Joyce and I considered drinking it until the pink elephants appeared. But the desperation of our situation and the knowledge of a certain monstrous hangover finished that thought.

Richmond suggested coming down for the upcoming tests, but once again I declined his offer. I took the big blow alone—we needed his business to continue operating, especially with the upcoming doctor bills. We resumed our old roles. Mine was at the hospital with Kyle; Richmond's was home with Anna and running his business.

Watching the bone marrow and bone biopsy made me nearly vomit. Seeing Dr. Mogul bear down on the needle with the screwing motion necessary to extract the bone for biopsy was intense. Even though Kyle was sedated, he squirmed during the harsh procedure. Dr. Hartman explained the tumor was on the right side of the rectum. He planned on a back-entrance incision—up the crack of Kyle's rear end. Or it would be the "baby fillet."

Instead of our planned celebration for Kyle's first birthday, we were preparing him for pre-op, surgery and recovery—an inpatient stay of five to 10 days. Instead of birthday cake and punch, there would be clear liquid and antibiotics. Instead of a party hat, Kyle was looking at getting another Hickman tube.

He was still too little to know or care, which was a blessing. I drove Kyle back to Reno, carrying cases of champagne in the truck. I felt foggy, my brain trying to erase information too painful to hold. Clouded in dread, I pulled up in front of our house. Richmond and Anna came out and smothered us in hugs and kisses. I wrapped my arms around my family and held on to them for dear life.

We only had three days together. Then Kyle and I would go down for the two days of pre-op by ourselves. Richmond and Anna would come down the day before surgery and stay as long as I needed them. Robin, my best friend, was flying in from Chicago the day before surgery and would stay after Richmond left.

We felt as strong as we could under the circumstances and were incredibly thankful that we had had a few months off to regroup. We gathered our strength, knowing we would need all the reserves available to make it through the next few months.

Our families were terribly afraid that we were going to lose Kyle to cancer. There were a lot of long-distance phone calls and lots of local family support. We gathered around each other trying to make sense of it all. Lots of prayers were said and tears flowed. We had done this once before; but this time was much different. We knew kids who had died or were going to die. Death was no longer such a stranger.

THE FIRST TIME AROUND, I thought if we did everything we were supposed to, Kyle would be fine; after all, Dr. Hartman told us there was a 90 percent chance of recovery. This time, I wasn't so sure. The statistics also were much different. Dr. Carolyn Russo, the attending physician overseeing our case, told us she only had stats on four or five children in the country whose tumors had acted like Kyle's. She didn't fill us in on the current status of those particular cases. It was hard to feel safe with that small of a data base. She still felt Kyle had a "good chance of long-term survival." What did *that* mean?! Long term...one year, five years, 60 years? Unfortunately, there wasn't an answer to my question.

The world of oncology scared the hell out of me and I didn't want to return to it. But here I was. I could handle the surgery, because it was only one day. But we were facing months of chemo, fever and neutropenia, and being separated from our family, all over again. I felt we were going back to hell.

A smaller frustration was that the new Children's Hospital had moved its opening date back. The new facility was named the Lucile Salter Packard Children's Hospital at Stanford (LPCH@S). There, the regular pediatrics unit (Peds), Peds Intensive Care Unit (PICU) and the oncology unit would all be in the same building instead of spread out at different facilities, as at the current facilities. We had already seen the hi-tech facility at the grand opening celebration in April. It was luxurious compared to the old units. Each room in the cancer ward had a day bed with a small overhead reading light, allowing a parent to stretch out or sleep comfortably bedside. The rooms overlooked roof-top gardens with benches for enjoying fresh air and sunshine. I called the new hospital, "Lucy's Hyatt." Each room was fitted for one or two patients, instead of three or four, and had its own bathroom. It would provide as much comfort as possible under trying circumstances. Until LPCH@S was open the old Peds unit—which I referred to as "Ghetto Peds"—would suffice.

Kyle and I drove back to Stanford on a crystalline clear day. We passed through the Sierra Nevada and reveled in God's handiwork. The California foothills are so graceful with their golden grasses blowing in the breeze. The enormous bridges that cross San Francisco Bay still astound me. Mother Nature and man's accomplishments left me awe-struck. I never tired of that journey.

I just hoped man and God could work together again, so we could spend more days or even years with our son. Kyle was so joyful all the time, we just didn't want to lose that happiness.

We didn't want to lose our Smiley Kylie.

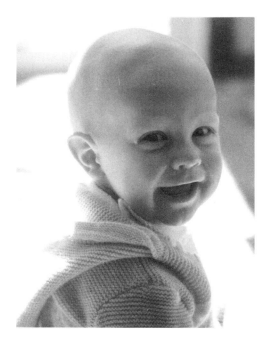

Kyle when he was completely bald in January of 1991.

Kyle with his I.V. hat during group #1 of chemo in January, 1991.

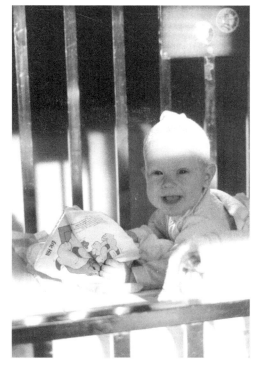

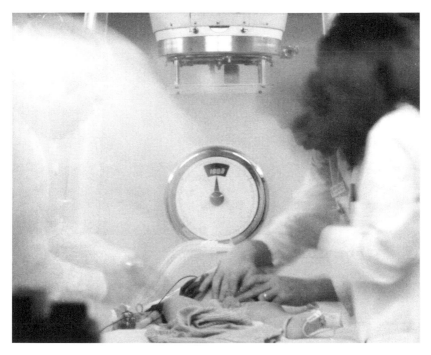

Radiation therapy setup, as everyone scurries around Kyle, who is already under a general anesthetic. During actual treatment, the door slams shut with all others safely on the other side of the door.

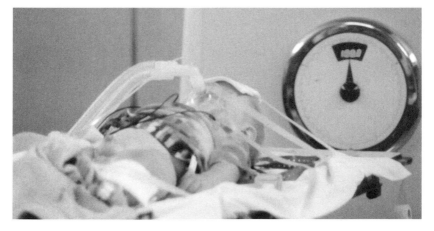

Kyle under a general anesthetic at set-up for his daily radiation treatments.

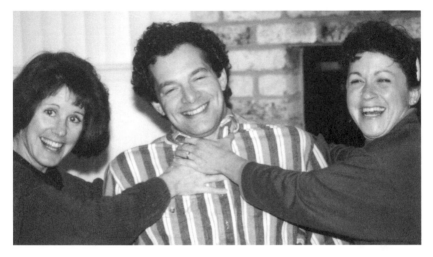

Drs. Kim and Jim Stone (with Donna) at our home away from home. We teased that Jim had two wives—poor guy!

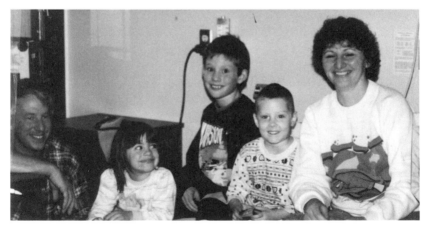

The Lupro family at Children's Hospital at Stanford in the Day Hospital. (Left to right) Bob, Nicole, Tyson, Cassie and Joyce.

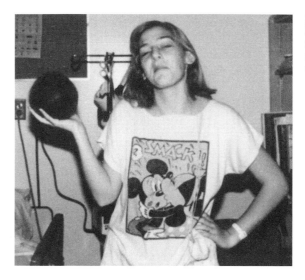

Kendra Green with her hairball "that freaked out the new residents" in October of 1990.

Kendra Green (in Santa hat) with her Mom and Dad (Sharon and David) at the Christmas Doobie Brothers Concert at Children's Hospital in the cafeteria, 1990.

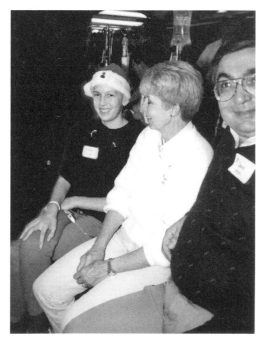

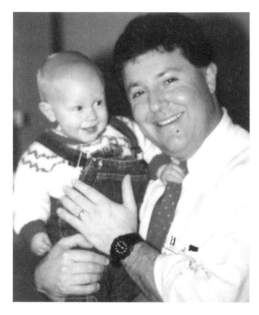

Dr. Mark Mogul holding Kyle in February of 1991.

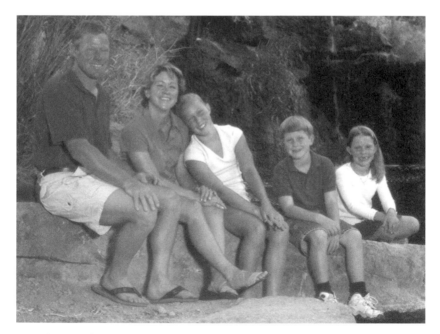

(Left to right) Richmond, Donna, Anna, Kyle and Haley Breen in Reno, Nevada, 2000.

CHAPTER 11

ANOTHER MAJOR SURGERY

So, once again, we found ourselves checking in at Stanford for surgery. *Sign here, fill this in, fill that in, sign there.* I could have wallpapered Kyle's room with all our admit slips except our copy was always pink instead of blue.

The pediatric ward was old, with less room built in for cots to accommodate parents who wanted to sleep near their children. Sleeping bedside wasn't a choice, so I got the nurses' station phone number and the direct line to Kyle's room. He was in his crib just idling. Oral antibiotics and Jell-O were the only items on his agenda. I would wait and get dinner on the way back to Kim and Jim's. I felt it would be cruel to eat in front of Kyle when he wasn't allowed a real meal. He didn't seem upset about being at the hospital, though I was still filled with fear.

The next day, Kyle's regimen called for Jell-O only, and "N.P.O." after midnight. N.P.O. meant nothing to eat or drink. Kyle was scheduled for surgery at 9:45 a.m. Wednesday, May 29, and they wanted his stomach completely empty so if he threw up while under a general anesthetic he wouldn't have anything to choke on. Standard procedure. He didn't seem bothered by not eating, which was a relief.

That afternoon, Richmond and Anna arrived. We spent the afternoon and evening bedside with Kyle. After tucking him in, we went back to Kim and Jim's, a.k.a. Kimberly and Jim Bob, a.k.a. Jimberly and Kim Bob. We needed a good night's sleep.

The next morning we arrived at the hospital and waited to accompany Kyle to pre-op. The hospital staff was wonderful about including Anna. We went down the hallway to pre-op, where we all gowned up—booties, poofy hats, the works. Anna, only 3, wasn't quite sure about the hat, but the pre-op nurse explained to her that it was the only way they could let her in. We sat on a blanket on the floor, where the nurse poured out some blocks for Anna and Kyle to play with. We had the camera running to document pre-op. Kyle's IV was running. The tube was in his foot but he wasn't walking, so it really didn't matter. More IVs would be added later in surgery. They also expected to give Kyle a Hickman catheter. All meds and blood draws could be done via the Hickman, and that would provide tremendous relief. The countless needle jabs were taking their toll on Kyle's veins and psyche. His veins were scarred, making a clean IV start very difficult. Knowing he had no memory at this age helped make me feel better; but all the pokes left me mentally exhausted.

As Kyle was taken into surgery, we all tearfully said good-bye and gave him kisses. We went to the cafeteria to eat and kill time, trying all the while to ignore the remote possibility that he would-n't come out of surgery at all. If I had taken the time to consider what might have lain ahead, I would have fallen apart. It was too much to deal with, so I concentrated on keeping Anna busy. Richmond went for a run as he had during Kyle's first surgery. Again, it took about 10 miles for him to tire his body out. Anna and I were at the waiting area when he returned.

We were silenced by fear, by waiting through the unknown. I prayed it was a benign mass and not neuroblastoma. Dr. Hartman would do a frozen section of the mass right in the operating room which might—or might not—tell what we were dealing with. It would take a few days to receive solid results.

Finally, at 1:30 p.m., Dr. Schocat appeared. He and Dr. Hartman were a team. While Hartman tied things up, Schocat came out to give us an update.

Kyle had come through surgery with flying colors. They only had to perform a rear incision, removing his tailbone to access the tumor. The tumor was totally encapsulated, meaning it hadn't spread yet. That was fantastic. Kyle now had a Hickman in place.

Schocat paused. There was something else he had to say.

"Freeze pathology shows neuroblastoma," he said.

"Oh my God!" I gasped.

I felt as if I had been hit with a baseball bat. I started crying. Dr. Schocat was still talking as I started walking down the corridor, terrified and sobbing uncontrollably.

Richmond grabbed and held me. "We'll get through this," he said. "We'll be O.K....calm down Donna. We'll get through this."

I couldn't believe it. It was my worst nightmare. I wanted to run, to scream. I didn't want to be there anymore!

Richmond and I sat down with Anna and finally tried to absorb the information. We were every bit as stunned as the day we'd found out Kyle had cancer. I kept reflecting on how good it was that we had had a few months to gain some of our strength back before crashing back into the world of cancer.

Gradually the minutes passed, and I calmed down. We awaited Kyle's return to the ICU. He would be in recovery for several hours.

My dear friend Robin Shannon would be arriving from Chicago. I waited with Anna while Richmond picked her up at the San Jose airport. Later we all gathered in the waiting area. Kyle was wheeled through to Pediatric ICU (PICU) and hooked up to the various machines to monitor his overall condition. He was totally "tubular," teeming with lines going every which way. His wrists and ankles were tied down so he would stay on his stomach and not roll around. It was sad not to be able to hold or feed him. Seeing him connected to so many tubes was heartbreaking. In PICU visitation was limited, and once again they let Anna go in for a few minutes with Richmond or myself. The nurses were wonderful and gave us a phone number so we could go across the street for dinner, call in to check, and try to relax as much as possible.

That night, Robin stayed in an inexpensive motel. Richmond, Anna and I stayed at Kim and Jim's. We didn't want to take over the Stone's home any more than we already had. We agreed that once Anna and Richmond were back in Reno, Robin would join me at the "Wilke Way Resort."

The next morning, we picked up Robin at her less-than-optimal sleeping accommodations, and off we went to the hospital for the morning update. I felt purged of my grief and shock from the day before. As I noted in my journal: "We know we can do this as we've done it before." Still, a lot of the time spent at the hospital those first few days after Kyle's second surgery were a fog. I was clouded in emotion. I kept asking myself, "How could I have been so incredibly stupid?" To think that we were home-free and the lucky ones. I kept beating myself over the head with the question, "Who the hell did I think we were?" I was consumed by bitterness.

That afternoon, Robin, Anna, Richmond and I were walking on the Stanford grounds. While we passed in a crosswalk, a car came to a stop perhaps a trifle close to us, and I remember being so filled with rage that I had to quash an impulse to leap onto the hood of the car and punch the windshield until it shattered so I could beat the hell out of the driver within.

I was on the edge, snarling at Anna, being a total bitch to Richmond and probably less than pleasant to Robin. They tried to reason with me. Richmond calmly said, "You have got to get a grip on yourself and deal with your anger."

Anger! Wow, was I angry. If some degenerate would have crossed me on one of those first days of Kyle's relapse, I probably would have just obliterated him with karate punches and kicks and spat on his crumpled body without a second thought. That was exactly what I wanted to do to cancer. But I couldn't find it to pummel it. It was intangible—an impossible opponent. Five years of kempo karate and a third-degree brown belt wouldn't help me hit something I couldn't see.

That evening, we went out for pizza after saying good-night to Kyle. Still throbbing with anger, I was unbelievably difficult to be around. I was seeing too much red to be able to acknowledge my feelings. Anger overshadowed my every thought and deed; I snapped at everyone within striking distance. After a stress-filled dinner, Richmond was still trying to make progress with me. Robin had taken Anna out for a walk. Anna was antsy. After a long wait for her dinner she had started getting squirmy and impatient after finishing her meal. Robin hoped that taking Anna outside would make it easier to work the problem out.

Finally, the light bulb lit up in my head. I was furious with myself. Having seen enough at Children's to know there were no guarantees, I had still showed up for Kyle's checkup with a nonchalant, happy-go-lucky attitude, as if we were somehow beyond the long tentacles of cancer. I had stood there grinning naively like an idiot—until the bad news was delivered. My personal disgust was stronger than any I had experienced. And the source of my disgust was myself—my foolhardiness. I now knew I would never be lured into such complacence again. I couldn't afford to set myself up like that. It would be better to be cautiously optimistic.

Now that I understood where my anger had come from, I felt much better. Drained both mentally and physically, I looked forward to a good night's rest.

Richmond was supposed to be leaving the next day, though he considered staying an extra day due to my mental state. He was probably afraid I'd knock the heck out of some poor unsuspecting fool who offended me by accident. But the next morning I began the day with a fresh attitude. *We could get through this, and we would.* We went to the hospital to see Kyle and get an update. While there, I found out that when a nurse was removing a main artery IV, Kyle had moved and it flicked toward her, splashing blood. I overheard her talking to a doctor about it.

"What does, 'being splashed' mean?" I asked.

"When I was taking out his arterial IV, some blood splashed in my eye," she said.

I urgently replied, "You're going to test him for AIDS, aren't you?"

"We can only do that with a signed consent form and I really only worry if they've had a number of transfusions," she said.

"He's had about 24 transfusions," I said. "Get the consent form. I'll sign it."

I was stunned. Here were people fighting to save lives, and they were barely able to protect themselves. I believe any health-care worker who is put in jeopardy has a right to know what he or she is up against. We owe them that respect.

KYLE WAS DOING GREAT for a kid who had just had his rear end bisected, and we were all feeling a lot better about trying to survive Round Two in the cancer war. Richmond and Anna would stay the day and leave in the morning. I felt solid and Robin was there to baby-sit me. She could sit with Kyle some of the time.

The next morning, we went back to the hospital and Richmond and Anna said good-bye to Kyle. I gave them both big hugs and reassured them I was fine and that going home was a good idea. So off they went to the home front. Robin and I spent another long day in the hospital taking turns sitting with Kyle and talking to each other.

It was incredibly soothing to have her there. Not only were we the best of friends, but she was a nurse, so once again I was relieved of providing explanations about tests and results. She knew the score and that's why she was there. It wasn't easy for her to drop everything and fly out West. She and her husband, Dr. Jay Shannon, had two boys and Jay was always on call. His specialty was internal medicine. They knew how serious our situation was and that Robin's support would be indispensable. Not only was being with Robin good for my sanity, but we planned on having a good time. Stanford Medical Center wasn't a resort, but Robin and I were quite creative.

We were busy making plans to enjoy Dr. Mogul's pool just two blocks from the front door of the hospital when we were informed that Kyle was to have his first meal that evening. His intestines were functioning, so I could start feeding my sweet baby. I was thrilled.

It was so encouraging to see him eat and take a bottle. He was as smiley as ever, displaying his ever-glowing warmth. He was such a delightful baby. His good nature amazed nearly everyone who came in contact with him. Robin and I stayed until Kyle finished his dinner and we put him "to bed" at 7 p.m., as usual. Richmond and I had never developed some of the lengthy bedtime rituals we had heard about from other parents. A story, a drink of water and some hugs and kisses were all our children needed. We didn't deviate from our normal routine because Kyle was in the hospital. He would go to sleep with no fuss.

We were going out! There was a terrific Cajun restaurant in downtown Palo Alto. It had a great wine list, broiled crawdads, awesome spicy oysters and delightful entrées. Just walking out of the hospital into fresh air was invigorating. My anger had subsided and I felt confident we could meet the challenge facing our family. I was ready to relax for the evening.

We got to the Suburban, hopped in—and there waiting for me was a note from my sweetheart.

I love you. You are very strong!

My heart and spirit are with you and for you.

If you need me, just call and I will be down in a moment.

You are the Best and a Super Mom!

See you soon. I love you.

I smiled and tried to start the engine. It didn't turn over. It was 7:30 p.m. and had been a long day; we didn't appreciate this hassle. Luckily, AAA was just a phone call away. The man who responded was helpful, saying he could start the car but we needed a new battery. We went to the auto center he recommended. The mechanic's response to our problem was simple.

"Sorry," he said, "but we're just getting ready to close the doors."

I just sank.

"Listen," I said, "my kid has cancer. He's just had surgery and I'm from out of town. Please…please take care of my car tonight."

"Oh my God," he replied. Well…yeah, OK."

Once in awhile it was all right to just lay it on the line.

Finally, Robin and I were off to dinner. Some of the wind was out of our sails, but we bounced back quickly. Laughter was a great restorative and we did our fair share that night. We carried on like a couple of college girls after exams were over. Therapy-shopping was on the roster for the following day. I needed new sunglasses so we could bask in the sun by Dr. Mogully's pool and be hip.

After a glorious dinner, we went back to Kim and Jim's to get some sleep before resuming hospital duty the following morning. I missed being able to sleep bedside with Kyle. It felt strange to be across town from my baby.

The next morning, Kyle was doing well, though still a bit lethargic. When he went down for a nap, Robin and I ran across the street to go shopping. I bought some sunglasses exactly like hers. Robin thought that was pretty amusing. "You just want to be as cool as me," she said. Then I looked for a new purse. I needed a bigger one for all the new hospital paraphernalia I would need everywhere I went. Kyle's Hickman would require a lot of care. There it was, the perfect purse—and exactly like Robin's! She just cracked up.

"You'll never be as cool as me. Ha!" she said.

We laughed about my purchases most of the way back to the hospital. We fed Kyle lunch and hung out with him until his afternoon nap. It was fantastic having Robin there. We had been close friends for more than 20 years and had been through many milestones together. First boyfriends, college, marriage, losing family members, having babies only a few months apart. We couldn't have been closer.

Kyle loved playing with Robin. She brought him an unbreakable baby mirror. They sat together with her saying, "Who is that baby in the mirror?" Kyle would smile and chuckle. They were quite the pair. I'm sure she was exhausted when she left, but I really appreciated the emotional support.

After Kyle went down for his afternoon nap, we went to Dr. Mark's pool. What a great hour of relaxation that was. Dr. Mark and his wife, Dr. Robin, who was equally nice, gave us a key to the pool entrance and told us to enjoy. Basking in the sun and fresh air was so intoxicating. The hour did us both so much good.

We wandered back to the hospital and wished we could have just hung out at the pool all day. However, it was back to reality and the work at hand. Kyle was his same charming self when we returned to the hospital. We stayed until his dinner and bedtime routine were over. Kyle was hooked to his Hickman. Finally, permanent IV access. No more pokes. Yahoo! I was relieved, though the added complications of caring for a Hickman were significant and a certain amount of caution would be necessary.

The tube was about 6 inches long where it came out of his chest. The remainder went under his skin, down a vein and into his heart. There was a cap on the end hanging out of his chest so a needle could inject various medications. The tube was taped to his chest so it wouldn't be pulled on. I had never watched anyone do Hickman care, though I had been in the same room and noticed that there were lots of solutions, sterile pads and Q-Tips involved.

The next morning, a nurse sent me to Children's, where they

were going to teach me Hickman care. Robin stayed and played with Kyle. I was sweating, I was so nervous. It was critical that the site stay as dry and sterile as much as possible. Kyle was only 12 months old, and drooled constantly due to teething. I was thrilled he wasn't going to get poked anymore, but the tube coming out of his chest made me very anxious. I opened my notebook to take notes.

Oh boy, there I was, roped into a whole new concept. *Sterility!* The nurse showed me how to open the sterile barriers without touching anything other than two tiny edges. It was a paper, about 16 inches by 24 inches, where all the other items were to be placed for the procedure. Nothing—not even my fingertips—could touch those edges or they would no longer be sterile. I was taught how to open all the various packages without touching the contents and keeping them where I needed them on the piece of paper called the "sterile field." There were Q-Tips on long sticks that came two to a package. Alcohol wipes were the hardest to get out of the packages without touching them. The wipes are wet and the interior of the small package is similar to foil to prevent them from falling out. The nurse taught me the various steps, using a doll with a Hickman attached. I only had to start completely over one time for wrecking the sterile field.

I was quite nervous, and the information I needed to absorb was just beginning. I took detailed notes:

For Heparin Lock Keep heparin in frig. always betadine wash the top of the lid, wait 2 minutes to let the betadine work. (kills germs) Draw 2 1/2 cc's of heparin in syringe for a 2 cc flush.—CHECK FOR AIR

To change cap

1. *Clamp off first, then betadine at junction. Leave betadine on 2 minutes then alcohol off.*

2. *Clean the heparin container with alcohol.*

3. *Fill 3 cc's syringe to 2 1/2 cc. Tap out air bubbles. NO AIR.*

4. *Open new cap*

5. *Fill cap with heparin—no air*

6. *CLAMP OFF*

7. *Remove old cap.*

   8. Put on new cap.

   9. Unclamp.

   10. Flush with 2 cc's continuing as removing needle.

   11. Tape the loop of Hickman tube and leave unclamped.
   When bathing Kyle cover entire site with a tegaderm patch.

OK, so that was changing a cap. Changing the dressing on Kyle's Hickman would take about 25 steps. The doll was hard enough to perform this on—she didn't even move. I could see I would need someone to hold Kyle flat on his back to accomplish this circus act.

Everything had to be laid out on the sterile field, then I would have to take Kyle's old dressing off. On the sterile field were two sterile urine specimen containers, one holding betadine and the other hydrogen peroxide, each with four Q-Tips, two gauze pads, four alcohol wipes and a dab of betadine ointment. I would apply these in order, starting around the opening where the tube came out of the skin and traveling in a circular motion so that I ended up farthest away from the actual opening. First were the Q-Tips dipped in betadine, which required a two-minute wait for it to do its stuff. After all those germs were dead, then came a circular cleansing with Q-Tips dipped in hydrogen peroxide. Then alcohol wipes closest to the site toward the outside, so that the germs that could be left would be moved farther from the actual site. After all the cleansing was completed, a drop of "betadine goo" was set at the site with another sterile Q-tip. Two sterile 2-by-2-inch gauze pads were laid by the tube followed by a 4-by-4-inch sterile gauze pad with tape to keep everything in place. As tempting as it was to tape the heck out of it so our 1-year-old wouldn't pull out this great new toy, the tape was also hard on Kyle's skin, leaving it red and irritated.

Whatever happened to just changing a cartoon Band-Aid? This was quite a challenge, without even considering the possibility of contaminating the sterile field and having to start all over. Concentration was a requirement, *not* an option, for this project.

I tried to absorb all the information that morning and was feeling pretty good with some encouragement from the nurse. I knew all the nurses very well by now and believed they would be upbeat yet honest with me. She said she was sure I would do fine. I felt like a surgeon washing up for the operating room. *Wash well, rinse fingertips up, don't touch anything.* Boy, I had a whole new view on germs. Between Hickman care and fever and neutropenia, I viewed everything I touched differently. Clean was one thing; sterile was a whole different ball game!

ROBIN AND I WENT to Stanford the next morning. Kyle was as cheerful as ever. Wow, he was one happy kid. I had to make out a list of necessary Hickman supplies for our home. Our medicine cabinet was sure going to take on a new look. The old look was aspirin, Children's Tylenol, Band-Aids, nail clippers. Whew…we were breaking into the totally prepared hospital look, carrying sterile units.

As I prepared to do Hickman care on Kyle for the first time, the pediatric nurse at Peds B was watching and Robin was holding (if memory serves; in retrospect, it may have been the other way around). I prepared my sterile field with all the appropriate paraphernalia for our opening act. There was so much to it, it did feel almost like a circus act. My nerves were frazzled and I felt as though everything was riding on my performance. Thinking through every step was essential; my total concentration slowly but surely carried me through the process.

It was time for Robin to return to her family. I would only be at the hospital with Kyle for a few more days and we could certainly manage that alone. My time with Robin over the past five days had been of value untold and truly carried us through more milestones. She was a true friend.

The doctors had decided Kyle would begin chemo in just a few days. The fourth and last round would coincide with the radiation. I wasn't quite sure what radiation was all about, but in a short time I would find out.

Then the doctor
came in to
the room

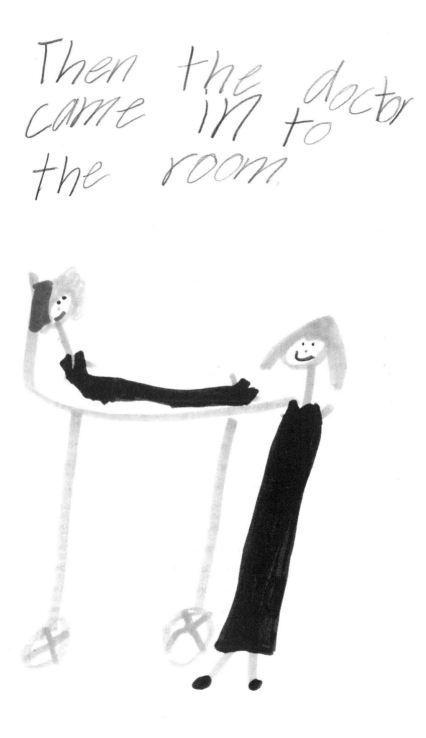

CHAPTER 12

LUCILE SALTER PACKARD CHILDREN'S HOSPITAL

Lucile Salter Packard Children's Hospital at Stanford was up and running. Ready for business. Hallelujah! I had already dubbed it, "Lucy's Hyatt." The story was that Lucile S. Packard gave $60 million to build the hospital to help children. Lucile Packard—"Lu" to her husband and friends—had devoted years of tireless effort to many children's causes. Except for a three-year absence while her husband served in Washington, D.C., as a deputy secretary of defense, Mrs. Packard was a member of the board of Children's Hospital at Stanford from 1967 (when it was still called the Stanford Home for Convalescent Children) until her death in 1987. For a year prior to her death, she chaired the transitional "new hospital" board responsible for the intricate planning and decision-making that led to this exceptional facility. It was Lucile Packard, according to board colleagues, who insisted that the windows in the new hospital be extra-large. She thought the children should be able to look at trees and grass and sky from their rooms and see people and flora in the hospital's interior courtyards. I was thrilled to be "checking into" the new luxury accommodations.

I was also a businesswoman, and familiar enough with new-business openings to know that no one would know where anything was located. A multimillion-dollar facility can't be moved overnight and have everything run smoothly. Even finding toilet paper might be tough. In Kyle's case I was going to have to locate diapers.

The day we checked into the new hospital, I chuckled because everyone was trying to locate this or that and it was almost impossible. Chaos ruled. The nurses appreciated my patience and understanding and perhaps my laughter at their expense. I knew in a few days things would be running much more smoothly.

A crew from CBS Evening News was on hand to cover the opening day. Each room had a huge teddy bear for the child to take home, and a poster depicting two children and a dog riding on the back of a huge cat. Each patient received a hot pink T-shirt that read, "I opened the doors." It was very exciting to be there at the opening. Kyle actually appeared on a two-second blip of the newscast, standing in his crib wearing the same smile he carried everywhere he went.

By this time I was an old hand at his Hickman care. I'd brought all my own supplies so I wouldn't have to locate anything on opening day. It was fabulous being in the new hospital with all its amenities. It more than made up for a few days of disorganization. Ours was a single room with our own bathroom—very uptown. There was a couch-type day bed with cushions on the back and a small overhead reading light. The window had a beautiful wooden blind that could be rolled with a handle crank from side to side. It was very nice—except for one detail: we were there to get Kyle his chemo.

We were starting a whole new protocol and the drugs were the "big guns." The side-effects might be much more severe, including the possibilities of kidney damage and serious hearing loss. They couldn't tell us for sure, as before, but I was prepared for the worst.

That morning, we had an appointment for Kyle to see Dr. Sarah Donaldson, one of the Stanford Medical Center radiologists. She had a fantastic reputation and was very nice. Kyle was to get 150 to 180 doses of radiation—"rads"—per day, for a total of about 4,000 over the month. There was a 10 percent chance it would render him sterile: the photon radiation energy disrupts the DNA of the tumor. As my journal entry read:

Cisplatin (one of Kyle's chemos) and radiation done together have a better tumor-killing power, than done separately. Radiation can aid in the maturation of tumors. No clear cut answers. Cytoxan (the first round of chemo) affects reproductive tissue. The radiation area would be marked with actual tattoo dots after numerous tests were done to ensure the area radiated was what they wanted. It would be near growth plates in his hips. "The growth plates will probably be avoided." (Possible) significant side effects—growth problems, sterility, small chance of leukemia, melanoma (skin cancer) where the radiation would be done. Cisplatin (chemo) can cause significant hearing loss and most always does some damage. Adriamycin (1st chemo) can do heart damage that may not show up until much later in life. Kidney damage was also possible.

This was tough information to take; not a pretty picture. But we had to try something and this was our best shot. These were some of the leading researchers at the hospital and they had worked with an entire network of doctors in the pediatric oncology group. The information went cross-country, with data compiled to give everyone the best fighting chance.

Richmond and I stopped Kyle's attending physician, Dr. Russo, one day and Richmond asked, "Do you have any medical papers I could read that are significant to Kyle's case? Or anything regarding the stats you gave us?" She said there was one paper she would find and copy for him, but that the cases weren't exactly alike. She reiterated, "There are only four or five children whom I know of whose tumors have reacted the same as Kyle's and have similar histories."

I visualized Kyle's upcoming chemo as the doctors aiming at a target while blindfolded. Maybe they would get it, maybe not. A lot of the information was very disturbing.

Kyle would be inpatient for three days of chemo, and for who knew how many more for fever and neutropenia. I couldn't imagine being in the hospital more than we had been before when he was getting Cytoxan and adriamycin. Having been gone from home more than 100 days from August through December, I was bracing myself for a brutal summer.

The night of Kyle's chemo, he didn't throw up much. The nurse gave him Reglan and Benadryl, which both combat nausea. It really helped, and he seemed to feel great the next day.

When we returned to Reno, we could see the worry on our family's faces though they were cloaked in smiles. The fear of losing Kyle consumed us all, making it hard to think about anything else.

On June 17, I took Kyle to Saint Mary's to get his blood counts checked. Fearing the worst, we waited for the results. But we were surprised. It was unbelievable. A week post-chemo, his counts were fantastic! We were elated and shocked, though we already knew the first round of chemo could be very misleading. A few rounds later, Kyle's little body might not be anywhere near as healthy. But we could hope.

We were enjoying our time home together. Debbie, Richmond's sister, my dad and Leigh all made tremendous efforts on Anna's part to try to make her feel special. Her trips to the park or ice cream parlor also gave Richmond and me time alone together. We had such a solid relationship and we would need it. The summer ahead would prove to be a time of great stress and fear.

A few more days went by. We went into the local lab for another blood draw. I had to bring all the Hickman paraphernalia to do a sterile blood draw. The hospital had all that was required, but it was more efficient and took a little of the stress off me when I brought my own supplies. I helped the lab at the hospital as I always had, only Kyle didn't have to be poked anymore. It was nice for everyone since he had always been such a hard poke. Once again, we braced ourselves for really low counts.

Another day with good counts! His body might not have reached the low period yet, but so far so good. We wished we could say the same for some of our friends.

Cassie was getting worse each passing day. The Lupros were trying to make the best of it. The Make A Wish Foundation is an organization whose primary goal is granting terminally ill children special requests. Make A Wish had sent the Lupros to Disneyland, where the family was well taken care of. Cassie was given a big button to wear. Bob can't remember what it said, but it translated into lots of extra attention from Mickey, Minnie and all the other characters who cruised the park.

Joyce and Bob were trying to keep her out of the hospital as much as possible. It soon became impossible. I felt as helpless as my family and friends felt about wanting to help us. The only thing I could do was continue giving moral support, instead of running when it got scary.

We weren't out of the woods ourselves, either, but everything is relative and Kyle was doing great. We went back to Saint Mary's one more time to get his blood levels checked.

He was on his way up. His counts astounded us. What, no transfusions? How could this be? We had weathered the entire month with no visits to a hospital other than blood draws. Dr. Mogul declared Kyle a trooper. He said to return for chemo on the first of July.

We relaxed as much as we could and continued with our daily life. Wake up, give Kyle an injection of heparin, have breakfast, give him oral antibiotic and much needed magnesium—a mineral which one of the chemos robbed his system of. Carry on and hope Kyle didn't throw up on any of us. Sometimes when he threw up, it just ejected out of his body, and there were no warnings because he was always so incredibly happy. He would just smile, puke, and smile some more.

I kept checking to see if his hair was falling out. I would gently tug on a tuft, so of course, Anna did the same. An older woman gave her quite the glance when Anna checked Kyle's hair status in the grocery store.

"I want to see if his hair's falling out," Anna responded. "He has cancer."

That poor woman didn't expect a 3-year-old to toss such information at her.

After grocery shopping I spent part of the afternoon reading to the kids, mostly Anna, but we all enjoyed the time together. Before dinner, we would get the Hickman care out of the way. It took about 30 minutes and was at the top of the stress list. To keep the field sterile during the 25 steps was challenging. Kyle lay nice and still and never fussed. Anna knew we couldn't stop what we were doing until the whole process was done. We changed the dressing every other day, more often if he got wet or dirty. After dinner and stories, we would inject his Hickman with heparin, and then: off to bed.

One night, Kyle was asleep and Anna was already in bed. Once she was in bed that was it—"no peeps," as I would say. Anna started calling us and calling us, much to our dismay. We were exhausted, as we were most nights by 7:30 or 8. I plodded up the stairs and was greeted by Anna.

"Mommy, you didn't hep-lock Kyle."

I stopped and thought, and realized she was right!

"Good girl," I said. "Thank you so much Anna. Good call!"

I went downstairs.

"What's up with Anna?" Richmond asked.

"We forgot to hep-lock Kyle," I said, "and our 3-year-old reminded us."

Heparin kept the blood from clotting and closing off the injection site. I don't know if missing one heparin lock would have done it, but we were very thankful that Anna was so sharp.

I WASN'T LOOKING FORWARD to being separated from Anna and Richmond during the end of the summer as Kyle's treatments intensified. For the time being we were so happy to do something as simple as sit at the dinner table and talk. Anna would chatter on about her dollies, playing outside or other things she felt her dad had missed during the day. Kyle just kept smiling, babbling baby talk with a few words like "mama" or "dada" interspersed. Watching him and Anna play together brought tears to our eyes on a regular basis, because as optimistic as we were, we knew those days might not last.

My thoughts constantly wandered to our friends at the hospital. Cassie was in terrible shape. I had also been on the phone with the Lindemanns, and Pat was also in bad shape. Both Cassie and Pat had T-cell Leukemia. Thomas wasn't in good shape either, along with many other children whom I had often seen, but never roomed with or gotten to know.

At least Kendra was doing well and keeping up her incredible attitude. This was reassuring. In a few days we would go back down to Children's to begin Round Two of chemo. Chemo could be cumulative, and we knew that Kyle might become much sicker as the treatment progressed. I often felt the sicker he became, the more the cancer was obliterated.

I knew he would probably lose his hair, but it was nevertheless distressing. Kyle looked somewhat normal unless you saw him naked or without a shirt. The Hickman projecting from his chest shattered any picture of normalcy. Kyle's hair would come out in tufts if given the slightest tug. Anna thought it was pretty entertaining when I kissed his head and it came off on my lips.

People would see Kyle and tell stories about their baby not having hair. I never said anything in return until one week at the grocery store. Twice in the same week, two separate people asked the exact same question and the second time around, I couldn't hold back.

A man thinking he was humorous said, "So, where did he get that Yul Brynner hairdo?"

"If you had five rounds of chemotherapy," I answered, "you wouldn't have any hair either."

The man returned my comment with a stunned look of embarrassment, muttering something unintelligible. That was toward the end of Kyle's first group of chemo. I was tired of people commenting on my baby's baldness.

As Kyle's hair continued to fall out, even he began to tug on it. The poor guy must have figured that if mommy and Anna were pulling on it, he should, too.

Kyle was constantly being bothered for something—medicine here, heparin lock there, Hickman care. We tried to do some "normal" things. While his counts were still up, we would go to the public pool at Idlewild Park in Reno.

To keep his Hickman dry, a tegaderm patch was used. It was like a large Band-Aid membrane that covered the whole area for bathing. Anna and Kyle loved the pool. They played together, splashing and laughing with an enthusiasm that helped push the fear back, if only for a short while.

It was time to pack our bags and go back to Children's Hospital for Round Two of chemo. We kept the good-byes very positive, and then Kyle and I hit the road. On the way down I always told him how great it was that we had chemo and all our wonderful friends at the hospital. These things were a gift.

The chemo was helping to save his life. The friends were helping to save our souls.

CHAPTER 13

CASSIE'S FINAL JOURNEY

Back to Lucy's Hyatt we went.

The first thing we did after arriving was check the board to see who our roommates would be. I had only met one mother and child who had proved so obnoxious that I pleaded with the nurses to put us in another room. Checking the board first would allow me to know what to expect if I knew the people.

We had a double-room this time with a mother and son who probably had enough problems without cancer in their lives. The mom and her boyfriend didn't seem to have a handle on the concept of moderation. Drugs and alcohol were a big part of their lives. They also fought a lot, and although they abstained from any screaming in our room, the tension ran high.

As a group, parents went to Pedro's for parent therapy, but we were always pretty conservative with our drinking. We all had talked about "drowning our sorrows," but knew life would only get more complicated by heavy drinking. There were a few children whose parents, I feared, had slipped over the edge. Cancer could do that to people.

The Lupros were all down from Alaska. Joyce's mom and dad lived about an hour from the hospital and Nicole and Tyson, Cassie's brother and sister, were at their grandma and grandpa's. As soon as Kyle and I were settled, I told the nurses I would be in Cassie's room. Kyle was happy and watched people walk by his window. I knew he would be fine, and the nurses knew how close we all were.

I walked into her room after giving a few knocks, and there were Bob and Joyce. I looked at Cassie's bed and was horrified. Her stomach was bloated so tight it shined. She was black and blue in some areas, her face bloated face and neck swollen. They had already been there a few days and knew Cassie couldn't last much longer. I went to hug Bob and Joyce and started crying.

"Great," I said, "this is just what you need, someone to visit and cry on you."

"We're just glad you're here," they replied.

I wanted to say something...anything...to help. There wasn't anything to say except, "I love you all...I'm so very sorry." We shared hugs and I filled them in on Kyle's medical status.

Most of that day, Bob or Joyce and I went for walks, talked about life, and death. They alternated leaving the room and I took each for a gin and tonic and something to eat. Cassie was dying, but sometimes children hung on for weeks. They would need some time out of the hospital if they were to stay sane. I checked on Kyle, but the nurses fed him, changed his diapers and took care of most of the duties I usually did. Kyle would be fine and was well cared for. The Lupros needed a friend more than ever.

Imagining what they were going through was impossible. Cassie had been so full of life and spunk. Her body was swollen beyond belief. Looking at her was looking at death. She barely breathed. I prayed for God to take her and let her run free of cancer and pain where there would be no more agony.

Sleep didn't come easy that night. Kyle was sick, due to his chemo, though not too bad, and my mind was having a hard time turning off.

The next morning, I showered and got myself together so I could go check on Cassie, Bob and Joyce. Cassie sounded even worse, her breathing labored, and was heavily tranquilized with morphine to kill the pain. I had never been in any situation that even remotely resembled this. Part of me wanted to run as fast as my feet would carry me, but part of me felt like I should offer to be with them all, *if* that was what they wanted.

"Do you want me here?" I asked. "The last thing I want to do is intrude, but if I can help in any way, I want to be here for you. We are good friends. I'm trusting you to tell me what's right for you."

"I want you to stay," Joyce said. "There will be a priest in later to do last rites if you want to be here."

Last rites were something I had only heard about. I wanted to tell Cassie I loved her and help bless her into a better world. The priest would be there in an hour or so. Bob and I went for a walk, talking about Cassie. She was in terrible pain with her body shutting down. At that point anyone who loved her would want her to rest in peace.

Bob asked a question that made me pause and contemplate.

"If they give her enough morphine, it can end her pain forever," he said. "What would you do if it were you?"

As I walked it occurred to me that I'd never been asked a more important question. Courage would mean telling him what was in my heart, what I believed I would have done under similar circumstances.

"I would up her morphine and let her go," I replied, hoping to God I was never faced with the same decision.

Bob told me they were thinking of taking a vacation after Cassie died. They had a van to drive back to Alaska. A few extra days to do something enjoyable would do everyone good. Tyson and Nicole spent the two previous years with their family separated and their sister dying. They deserved some time to try to have a little fun on their way home.

Bob asked me what I thought about vacationing after Cassie's death, because they had heard some opposing arguments.

"I think it's a great idea," I said. "You guys deserve it and if somebody doesn't like it, tough! That's their problem."

We also discussed the issue of burial or cremation. Bob had heard that some siblings of another child who had died of cancer were extremely upset when they found out the child's body had been burned. For that reason and others he thought they would bury Cassie in Juneau.

We were outside and had covered some incredibly serious subjects. We both felt the moment somehow lighten.

"If you cremated Cassie," I said, "you could take her on vacation with you." Bob just looked at me and laughed.

WE WENT BACK TO the hospital to spell Joyce. We talked about my being bedside and they both wanted me there. Joyce's parents came and we all said hello. They were a wonderful family and had opened their home to their children and grandchildren for what had stretched to about two years. This was not the way anyone wanted it to end. We were all sitting or standing around Cassie's bed when the priest said some prayers and anointed her with holy water.

Tears and sorrow filled Cassie's room that day. Part of me couldn't believe it was real. How could it be? All the praying in the world hadn't saved her and there couldn't have been more put forth on her behalf. I felt so vacant and flooded with sadness.

I went again to check on Kyle and spent some time with him. He was his usual happy self and pretty unaffected by what he was going through.

I called Richmond from the phone in Kyle's hospital room, and told him what the earlier part of the day had been like. Another priest was coming in a little while and I was going to join Cassie's family to offer what love and support I could.

Again, I asked Bob and Joyce if they wanted me to stay or go.

"I don't know how you can stand it," Bob replied, "but we want you to stay."

It was such a hard place to be, but it felt like the right thing to do. As we each said a prayer over Cassie, I thanked her for being such a joy in my life and told her how much I loved her. I wanted her to know how much she had touched my heart and soul. She knew we loved her dearly, but we had no way of knowing if she heard our words.

She was overtaken by cancer and her poor little body was frightening to look at. Her skin looked as though it was stretched so far that her shiny torso would just burst. It was hard to believe that this spunky little girl, who took rides on the IV pole while being pushed by her parents, was trapped in this horrible mass of flesh before me. I could still recognize her face, though it was very bloated. I prayed for God to end her misery.

That evening we were all exhausted. I offered to take Bob or Joyce, or both, across the street for dinner. Food was a necessity, and after some discussion we decided the three of us would run over for a quick bite. Thankfully, we were able to sit outside and get some fresh air. The hospital could be stifling and we were exhausted. We ate quickly, paid the bill and hurried back to the hospital.

Bob and Joyce glanced at me as we went toward our respective rooms. "I'm going to check on Kyle and give Richmond a quick call. I'll see you in a few minutes," I said.

Kyle slept in his crib while I lay on my bed and dialed up Richmond. Just after he answered, a nurse rushed in.

"Cassie just died," she said.

"Cassie died," I blurted into the phone. "I have to go. I'll call you back."

Richmond didn't catch what was said before the line disconnected. In fact, he worried until hours later when I called him back.

Running into their room, I found Bob and Joyce weeping. We hugged while we were all crying.

"Cassie Lou, I love you," I cried, hugging Cassie. "God bless you."

We were all sure that Cassie knew she was dying and had waited until Bob and Joyce were back from dinner. She had died a few minutes after they returned to her bedside. We were thankful that she was no longer in pain.

I took a few roses out of the arrangement in her room, laid one on her chest and took two home to dry and to remember her by. The tears continued and I was overwhelmed by a thought that wouldn't leave my mind. Not able to shake it, my sobbing continued. The question was so difficult, I could barely stand the thought.

"How are you going to be able to walk away…and just leave her?"

Joyce looked at me and tearfully replied, "I don't know."

It was so final. Her spirit was in a better place, but her body was still in front of us. My mind was having a terrible time trying to find places to put all this new information.

Cassie's nurse that evening was a young German woman who was usually quite reserved. She came in to unhook the IV's and the other medical paraphernalia. She lost her reticent demeanor and had a difficult time unhooking the IV line as the tears clouded her vision. She had dropped her guard and emotion flowed as she expressed her sympathy. The doctor followed to officially check Cassie's vitals and take care of the death certificate.

A few hours after Cassie died, Bob and Joyce were as ready as any two parents could ever be to walk out that door. Cassie's body was cool to the touch and I gave her one last kiss as we left the room to go to their van. I wished so badly that I had some words of wisdom, something to help ease their pain.

"I love you," I said, feeling inadequate. "If there is *anything* I can do for you—please let me know."

They both looked at me as Bob replied, "You've already done it... you were there for us."

I walked back into the hospital knowing they would never be back or be roommates again. I was sad for all of us. We would all miss Cassie so very much. She was an incredible little girl. We would also miss each other.

I returned to Kyle's room. He was fast asleep. I lay down on my bed to call Richmond. He was worried sick. All he had heard was my frantic voice and that I would call him back. It had been hours.

He was very relieved to know Kyle was OK. He also felt awful for the Lupros. We talked about how much cancer stinks and how grateful we were that Kyle seemed to be doing so well.

"I love you, sweetheart," I said before hanging up. "Have a good sleep."

Sleep came easy for me that night. Keeping my eyes open would have been nearly impossible: they were almost swollen shut.

CHAPTER 14

THE CANCER WAR CONTINUES

The next day I stayed by Kyle's bed, hugging him and praying for strength for all the children and their families. Pat Lindemann was also in terrible shape. He wasn't going to make it. T-Cell leukemia was awful. It made me angry, but I tried to stay focused on the beautiful little baby in front of me. Kyle was as charming as ever and when I cried it didn't seem to upset him. Kyle's IV dripped VP-16—a chemo drug— that morning, and later that day we drove home to Reno.

Going home was different this time. My life was changed by what I had seen and experienced. I felt pretty rough around the edges. I had only been gone from home three days, but it felt considerably longer.

Anna was glad to see her brother and excited because we were going to a Fourth of July party the next day. I couldn't imagine sitting at a party and wouldn't have considered it if it hadn't been family. We all looked battle-worn, but managed to put on smiles. I knew I would be asked how my week had been and I didn't feel like the truth was "appropriate party talk." The truth was our lives were filled with fear, anxiety and tension. Luckily, there also was love and support. Everyone tried to keep a happy face on for us, too, knowing that we didn't need to worry about how someone else felt about our situation.

Over the next few days I tried to get back on my feet, knowing that our lives had to go on. Anna was a grounding force of reality and would still need the customary books, lunch and loving that was a necessary part of her life. I took her to our local grocery store. Most of the clerks knew who Cassie was because of the store's donation for the Bone Marrow Drive. We gathered our groceries and went into line with a clerk we knew and waited our turn. As our groceries were rung up the gal inquired about my day. Anna said brightly to the clerk, "Cassie died, and now she has a brand-new pink bike up in heaven!" The woman stopped what she was doing and looked at me as if to say, "Is it true?"

Anna always made me smile. Her viewpoint often brought perspective that adults failed to see. She helped keep me focused. Had Kyle been our only child, I might not have coped as well.

I felt that my hospital friends needed support and I intended to give them as much as I could. The Lupros were at Joyce's mom and dad's house in San Jose, gathering their thoughts and belongings in preparation for the drive back to Alaska. We were all very happy to know they would be stopping in Reno on their trip north. We were safety nets for each other and explanations weren't necessary. Our time together could be spent enjoying each other's company. Anna was excited that Cassie's sister, Nicole, was coming, but at 3 years old was having a hard time understanding why Cassie wasn't. Cassie and Bob had stopped in Reno on one of their adventures and Anna and Cassie had jumped on beds like kangaroos, laughed and raced through the house.

I checked on the Lindemanns. They were taking Pat home. He didn't want to die in the hospital. He was in terrible shape and old enough to know what he wanted. They had offered one more type of experimental chemo and Pat had said, "No." He knew the pain that would be in store and the dim chances of a cure. At that point, they were only offering a few more months, if that.

As an adolescent, Pat was old enough to process the information and unwilling to be a player in the game anymore. He had suffered enough pain and expressed as much. His parents, Bill and Jackie, were wonderful people. They respected his wishes, leaving the hospital with morphine and hopes that their son would be as comfortable as possible. He was going home. It was what he wanted and the least they could do for him. I told them I would be thinking of them, and if they wanted to call, I would be happy to hear from them.

So far, Kyle seemed to be doing well with chemo. It was now seven days post-treatment, and time to get his blood drawn. We went down to Saint Mary's. The lab techs now only held Kyle while I performed the draw. I was more familiar with a Hickman and it made me more comfortable.

7/8/91 A.M. Blood Draw
W.B.C.—2.4

Bands—0

Platelets—364

Hemoglobin—10.9

Polys—41

ANC - 984

Thinking the counts were too good to be true, I called Dr. Mogul to ask if I should believe the figures."Enjoy it!" he said."He's doing great!" It was wonderful and we were thrilled. I was hoping Kyle and I would not be going down to Stanford at the same time the Lupros were coming to see us.

The next day, the Lupros arrived. We were all incredibly comfortable with one another. Tyson (the oldest) watched the younger kids play and enjoyed them as much as an older sibling does. Kyle was still only a year and a few months old, not walking yet but happy as could be. Nicole and Anna were two peas in a pod. We adults talked until the wee hours. There was nothing that couldn't be said—we had been through the worst. Still, it felt funny to do Hickman care for Kyle while the Lupros were there. Administering the daily heparin locks, antibiotics and magnesium tablets, were almost embarrassing because we were lucky enough to still have Kyle.

The morning the Lupros were getting ready to leave, I was doing Kyle's heparin lock. The fluid didn't travel through the tube properly and left a bubble. Not the administrative method we were shooting for (no pun intended). The fluid was caught in between the layers of the tube and hadn't traveled through the Hickman. I knew as soon as I saw it that Kyle and I would be going to Stanford to have the Hickman fixed. Joyce and Bob just grinned and said,"I'm so glad we don't have to worry about that anymore." Not glad that Cassie was gone—but a Hickman takes a lot of care, and everything associated with it is stressful. They were simply glad cancer was gone from their lives.

I wished Bob, Joyce, Tyson and Nicole a safe journey, with hopes that they had a little fun. They could all use it. I wondered if they knew how to have fun anymore. There were days I felt like I was seriously out of practice. I couldn't imagine being in their shoes. I called Stanford and was informed that the end of the Hickman could be cut off and another piece reattached. We were back on the road.

The next morning, Kyle and I jumped in the truck to come home. We would be back by late afternoon and I was looking forward to cooking my family dinner and relaxing! Kyle was easy, though his appetite was slight. His favorite meal was two eggs scrambled with ketchup. I used to laugh every time I made those for Kyle at Kim and Jim's. Jim really watched his cholesterol and though he said, "Anything you can get him to eat is good at this point." I knew the eggs must have made him cringe. Thoughts like that left me chuckling during the day. It was important to get the laughs where I could. Being easily amused was a definite plus during cancer duty.

I was thrilled with Kyle's blood counts, as were Anna and Richmond. Anna couldn't understand why Kyle wasn't getting any transfusions and occasionally would say, "Mom...I think Kyle looks pale, maybe we should have counts done." Indeed, we all felt like something should be done on an almost daily basis. After all, during the first group of chemo we were hardly ever home and the second group of chemo was supposed to be even harder on him. Why was he doing so well? We had daily duties, but we were at home (thank God) and Kyle's good condition started to make me nervous. Most of his hair hadn't fallen out. He only had about 1 strand out of 500, but he still had a little bit of hair. He was always happy—and that was constant. But those counts...why weren't they as low as before?

I tried not to worry and to concentrate on the good: enjoying our time together. We knew the end of the summer would leave us all separated for about four weeks. For the time being, we were enjoying the season. Anna checked on the progress of the garden on a daily basis. Kyle was still crawling everywhere. Richmond and I were thrilled to be able to hold each other every night. Life was as good as it could be under the circumstances. It was mid-July. The crickets began their soothing chirping every evening.

I DECIDED I BETTER keep in touch with the Lindemanns since my last call to them had them taking Pat home. I learned he had died July 9.

It was hard to believe that cancer had claimed another kid. Cassie and Pat both had T-Cell leukemia. Understanding how an adult whose body was abused would get cancer was easy; but these kids were so innocent. No matter how I looked at the facts, they didn't add up. Thankful that Pat was no longer in pain, I prayed for Bill, Jackie and their family to remain strong.

It was challenging to keep a positive attitude after hearing heart-wrenching news. And though I knew every disease was different (there are many factors just for neuroblastoma), I was terribly afraid. None of my friends who had lost children thought they would in the beginning. The whole idea of remission scared me. I continued to visualize people in remission walking around with the hatchet over their heads, hoping the guy with the huge shears wouldn't cut the string holding it. But now we were the ones hoping and praying for continued safety. Except—did anyone ever take away the hatchet?

All these ideas filtered through my thoughts, interrupted by various Disney books, videos, meals with my family and daily activities. My workload increased as I prepared as much as possible for the month of Kyle's radiation. With nine days remaining it looked as though we would escape fever and neutropenia again—amazing!

I stocked up on snacks, drinks, meat, paper goods, etc. Keeping busy was good for me. One of my coping mechanisms was to go, go, go…sleep…go, go, go,…sleep. It gave me less time to ruminate.

As the days passed, we were thrilled that Kyle's blood counts never dropped as they had with the first group of chemotherapy. I became increasingly depressed as our departure date approached. Richmond was encouraging, but I had dubbed the upcoming four weeks, "Hell Month." Kyle was going in for chemo, followed by daily doses of radiation, concluding with radiation and chemotherapy administered concurrently. Even Donna the Optimist couldn't see how Kyle's upcoming schedule could be anything other than a living hell.

The comfort of the new hospital and the wonderful location were helpful. The rooftops at Children's Hospital were pleasant, with gardens and pathways where we could catch a breath of fresh air. Hopping a gate out to a big open rooftop (I felt at home on the roof) was the beginning of my kempo karate workout. A "kata,"—a series of strikes, kicks, blocks and stances—called Tiger and Crane had about 600 moves. Visualizing "cancer" as my enemy, I got some great stress-relief through those workouts. It felt good to exercise and get my "ya-yas" out.

When Kyle received radiation only, we were outpatient, leaving the hospital after our morning appointment. I didn't want to impose on Kim and Jim anymore, but after we all discussed the situation, the decision to stay at their home was made. They must have been sick of us by that time. They were even buying a new house just a few miles from the hospital. I said they had to because we wouldn't go away. The move to "the Willow Road Resort" would happen by the end of July, providing us with separate bedroom and bathroom quarters. We would be very comfortable and planned on making every effort to simplify life for Kim and Jim.

Finally the day came for Kyle and me to leave for Stanford. Chemo Round Three would start on July 22 and there were tests to be done before radiation could begin.

"Are you sure you'll be OK?" Richmond asked again. "I'll be down the moment you want me—just call."

I had his support and felt confident, though it was cloaked in dread. I knew it was unrealistic for the whole family to spend an entire month at Stanford. Anna needed to sleep in her own bed, and Richmond's business was to keep the family financially afloat. We said our "I love you's," passed out hugs and kisses, and Kyle and I were on our way.

I was not looking forward to "Hell Month." On the drive to the Bay, all kinds of flowers were in bloom.

CHAPTER 15

HELL MONTH

Though imposing on people was difficult for me, getting over that hurdle was necessary. The Moguls opened their home to Kyle and me, and we were grateful. The Ronald McDonald House was under construction. When they finished both the remodeling and the addition of the one next to the hospital it would be a different story. Room availability at the temporary Ronald McDonald House also was a problem.

I was glad Kim had been honest the week of their move into their new home.

"You'll have to find somewhere else. I'm sorry," she'd said.

"Please don't apologize," I'd replied. "You and Jim have been so incredibly generous, I would hope that after all we've been through, if there's a bad day, week, or if you're sick of us, you'd be honest. I'm counting on that, Kim."

After staying at the Moguls' one night, it was time for Kyle and me to check into the hospital. First thing that morning, Kyle had an appointment down at XRT (X-ray Therapy). It was in Stanford Medical Center, down long winding hallways, and I ran pushing him in a stroller, checking the crossing corridors to make sure I wasn't going to crash into anybody. I often ran through the corridors, because I usually had to wait quite awhile during Kyle's tests or procedures. Kyle liked it when I pushed him fast. With the wind in what little hair he had, he would laugh and kick his feet as we cruised the corridors.

Our first morning at XRT they tattooed five dots on his body to mark the area to be radiated. The area was near his pelvic growth plates, critical to his development. His testicles would be wired together each day to keep them out of the field of radiation. Kyle would be put under a general anesthetic to ensure no movement whatsoever during the tattooing, and again each morning for his radiation therapy. This wasn't necessary for adults, but telling a 14-month-old to lie still obviously would not work. Hopefully, the general anesthetics wouldn't be too hard on him. Each morning I recorded what drugs were used and who the attending and resident anesthesiologists were. The more information I kept in my journal, the better I felt, knowing I was doing everything possible to keep abreast of the situation.

Sleep came easy. The next morning we needed to be at XRT by 8:30. Kyle was NPO (nothing to eat or drink) every night after midnight, until the next morning post-recovery from the general anesthetic. I put something for him to eat in my purse every morning—without his knowledge—so the minute he could eat, something would be available. Being NPO didn't seem to bother Kyle, but I didn't want him to wait any longer than necessary. I would sneak a quick bite to tide me over in the morning before we left.

We arrived at XRT and I was greeted by a terrific group of techs. Mike and Warren, Kiki and Maria would all be working on Kyle on a daily basis. They were very friendly and made me feel at home. I wanted to watch everything they did to him and learn what I could about his radiation treatments.

The day before Kyle's radiation began, they made a template out of an approximately 6-inch-thick piece of lead. Its purpose was to confine the radiation to a certain area. That made an impression on me. They wanted to do one more X-ray to make sure they would be radiating the correct area. The lead was cut precisely to the millimeter around his growth plates. If they missed, it could affect his height. I am 5-foot-2 and Richmond is 5-foot-6. I looked at Mike and Warren and said, "Hey...don't screw up, we have no room for error." They just chuckled and assured me proper placement wasn't a problem. I called the whole process "nuking," not realizing that nuclear medicine was a different department. They were polite and didn't correct me, enjoying my humor.

After the radiation was completed, Kyle was wheeled out of the XRT room. I followed the doctors who pushed Kyle's crib as he began to wake up from the general anesthetic. We went from XRT to the Post Anesthesia Care Unit (PACU), where he would be watched by nurses for an hour or longer, if necessary, until fully recovered from the anesthetic. Then we would go back to 2 North (the oncology unit). Other days when Kyle wasn't getting chemo, we would go back to Kim and Jim's. The XRT continued regardless of inpatient/outpatient status.

Kyle woke up from the anesthetic easily and had his customary smile within a few minutes. Halothane, the anesthetic, seemed OK for him. The nurses were immediately charmed by Kyle's sweet nature and I enjoyed meeting them. Seeing such a friendly group every morning for most of a month would be good for our morale.

By the end of the hour we were signed out and on our way to 2 North. Kyle's chemo had started so late the night before that I didn't get a good night's sleep and was going to nap as soon as possible. Our nurse checked on us and I inquired about Thomas, the boy in the room next door. Thomas had been our roommate on a number of occasions. He was a nice kid, about 12 or 13, and in bad shape.

Kathy, Kyle's nurse, said, "He's not doing well." In the real world that would mean he had the flu. In the realm of cancer, there was an entirely different translation.

"I'm going to check on Thomas as soon as I wake up from my nap," I said to Kathy.

She left to tend to other business and I fell asleep on my bed. Waking up relaxed and invigorated, I stretched and said hello to Kyle. Shaking off the sleep, I realized I needed to check on our old roomie. I got up and walked out into the hall and saw Kathy.

"Is this a good time to say hi to Thomas?"

Her eyes welled up with tears. "He just died a few minutes ago," she said.

"Oh my God," I cried. "How could I have waited?"

Kathy and I went into Kyle's room. We talked, cried together and hugged each other. I sobbed and rocked myself after she left. Thomas was the third child in three weeks to die. I couldn't fathom how this was possible. They were all such good kids—how could this be happening? Was God on vacation? Taking a really long nap? I was growing very angry. I cried some more, went out in the hall and paused as I saw Thomas' father. We didn't know each other. Though we had passed in the halls and said hello on occasion.

Looking at him with tears in my eyes, I whispered, "I'm so very sorry. I really...am so sorry."

I hugged him and then I walked back to Kyle's and my room and wept until I felt limp. I felt negligent having napped before my intended visit to Thomas. I would never get to see him again, and that made me heavy-hearted and angry.

It was impossible for me to look the other way, or pretend I didn't know what was going on in the room next door. We had our own problems, and as difficult as they were, knowing Thomas had just died made it clear that we were the lucky ones. Seeing Thomas' father made me wish there was something I could do to make the sadness disappear. Yet, all I could offer were a few kind words. It didn't feel like near enough. I felt sick with sadness.

Kyle's nurse, Kathy, came back awhile later to check on me as well as Kyle, and we talked about her future. We were going to lose her too, though not to cancer. She couldn't take it anymore. Cancer had worn her out. In two days she was hanging up her oncology nurse hat.

I burst into tears once again. She was a wonderful nurse, whose heart was always in her work. We would miss her a great deal.

THE NEXT MORNING, KYLE and I woke up to a new day. He would have an XRT first, and after he was out of recovery from the general anesthetic, chemo would follow. If all went well, he and I would pack up, check out of our "suite" and go to the Mogul's house to stay for the remainder of the week. My wish was granted—the chemo went well.

Mark and Robin Mogul were both wonderful people and doctors. Mark was full of humorous anecdotes and helped keep my spirits up. Robin had quite a few amusing tales herself and as I got to know her, I could see they were a great team. Robin was doing her residency in psychiatry at Stanford.

"Hey Mark," I'd say, "you realize Robin married you so she would have a permanent case study. After all, anyone who stays in oncology for years—by choice—has to be a little wacko."

It was good staying with them and once again I didn't need to explain any of the tests or results. We could enjoy each other's company and leave cancer behind for the day. Robin was a great cook. As we ate and sipped wine, I reflected on how fortunate I was to be there. Relaxing in a home, sharing stories and teasing each other was wonderful. Richmond was grateful that I had friends and conversation during the evening.

Kyle and I went on adventures that kept him stimulated and me in motion. I ran for exercise, pushing the stroller along. Kyle didn't have much energy but really enjoyed looking at the scenery whizzing by or going into shops full of interesting things to look at or smell.

Older kids getting chemo had different opinions about smells and tastes. Chemo messed with the taste buds and someone who normally loved chocolate might not be able to stand it. It was as if someone else's taste buds were in their body and they didn't know what might taste good. Kyle's appetite was so low he wasn't very interested in food at all, though he still enjoyed scrambled eggs with ketchup, and peanut butter and jelly.

Occasionally, we would go to Stanford Mall and sit outside the cafe, watching shoppers stroll by. It helped pass an hour, and some days the hours were hard to pass. We would wander over to the produce store or meat store. On days when we only had XRT, we often had the day to ourselves by 10 a.m. As nice as it was to be at the Mogul's or Kim and Jim Stone's, it wasn't home. The times were tough and sometimes I just felt discouraged and depressed.

We moved into the lush accommodations at the "Willow Road Resort." The Stones' new home was lovely, and again only a few miles from the hospital. Kyle, Richmond, Anna and I helped break in the new place that first weekend. I was so glad to see Anna and Richmond. It had been a long, stress-filled week and I needed their support. Kyle seemed happy, as always, and was very excited to see Richmond and Anna.

Saturday, Richmond and Jim bought a variety of plants. Everyone pitched in with the planting of herbs and flowers, enjoying the added fresh touches to the yard. Richmond's business was landscaping and we all had fun getting involved in the project.

Having someone to hold Kyle during Hickman care was a luxury for me. In Reno, Richmond always held, but in Palo Alto I had to be resourceful. Kyle had to lie flat while I worked off of a sterile field for about 20 minutes. A few days I waited for Kim or Jim to come home but often they were late or Kyle and I were asleep. One evening, I decided to try it by myself. I lay out the sterile field, and all the other required paraphernalia to do the job on the bathroom floor. It was my best choice, since betadine was one of the fluids used and being blood-red, most certainly stained. After my field was organized I lay Kyle on the bathroom rug. Instead of someone else holding him, I placed my left leg over his hip area with my foot holding his right arm. I held his left arm with my right foot, leaving my hands free. He was so used to being held down for this procedure that he never fussed.

It worked! I was pretty pleased with myself, though it must have looked like a circus act. Hickman care was challenging and left me thankful that the bandage only had to be changed every other day. I used the same hold for Kyle's twice-a-day heparin lock. My improvised method helped eliminate some of my stress.

Minimizing stress was one of the topics we talked about during Anna and Richmond's weekend visit. We wanted to do whatever possible to keep life simple. They had come down Saturday and planned on returning to Reno on Sunday. Driving five hours with a 3-year-old proved challenging enough. Doing two days back-to-back sounded awful. We decided to take Sunday to visit Bay area museums, go to the beach and out for dinner. Monday we would all go to XRT and see Kyle through his treatment before Richmond and Anna would drive home.

We drove to the museums in Golden Gate Park first and spent as much time as two small children allowed. We went to the Bierstadt exhibit at the DeYoung Museum. The paintings were full of vibrant colors depicting oceans, and valleys covered with flowers. Bierstadt's works were gorgeous. Richmond and I both loved the time spent surrounded by such beautiful art work. Anna and Kyle didn't find it as interesting as we did. We wandered out of the museum after stopping at the gift shop, letting each kid pick out a little souvenir. Hot dogs from the vendor out front—and we were on our way.

Thinking of Kyle's less-than-adequate immune system, I said to Richmond, "God, I hope these aren't scary hot dogs." We had an entirely new view on germs and how much they could complicate our lives. We were borderline germ-phobic. With Kyle's previous group of chemo, every germ seemed to latch onto him and we would have to go to the hospital to treat his fever and neutropenia. So far, we had escaped F&N with the second group of chemo drugs.

We went to the beach after our hot dog lunch and enjoyed the sand in our toes and the carefree feelings the surf gave us. The kids had a ball playing in the sand and water. Richmond and Anna would run back and forth as the waves came and went. It was beautiful watching them, and I snapped pictures as they ran holding hands. As we sat on the sand, I set the camera on a tripod to take what I thought might be our best—and possibly last—good family photo. Every moment together was a treasure. If the chemo/radiation didn't work, Kyle would never look better, feel better, or be happier. I wanted to freeze the moment.

Then they take
the plastic
Out

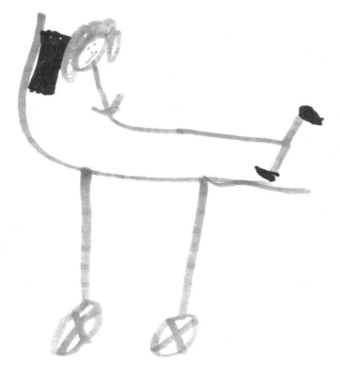

CHAPTER 16

HELL SUMMER CONTINUES

The next morning we arrived at XRT at our customary time, 8:30. As usual, I went into the radiation therapy room to talk to Kyle while he went under. Richmond and Anna waited outside, watching as Kyle was hooked up to various machines and monitors. I hooked up the oxygen monitor. This was a tiny red light attached to something like a Band-Aid. I wrapped it around his toe. Once in awhile someone else would hook it up, and often it was placed around the thumb he sucked. That really ticked him off; when he came out of the general anesthetic, he wanted to suck his thumb.

The most distressing part of XRT came after everything was hooked up. All details were double-checked, everybody left the room, and as the machine prepared to operate, a massive solid door slammed shut. The only one on the other side when the "nuke button" was pressed was our little baby. I *hated* that part, and it never got any easier. It was so dangerous, no normal person would want to be in the room; and yet there was our baby.

I understood as best I could the benefits of the procedure and explained them (again, as best I could) to Anna and Richmond as the 15-minute procedure ensued. Anna was fine with the whole thing; Richmond was another story. I don't know that anything would have made him feel OK about XRT.

The list of possible long-term side effects was much too lengthy. There was a small chance of leukemia and heart muscle problems due to the chemo. Hearing loss was a given and expected from the cisplatin chemo. The radiated area would be monitored for skin cancer, and Kyle's growth plates, which could affect the growth of his legs, were dangerously close to the radiation field. We would be alert for new tumors on Kyle's body for years. We found it necessary to push that information as far to the back of our minds as possible.

As Kyle finished treatment and we were leaving for PACU (Post Anesthesia Care Unit), Anna and Richmond got organized for their trip home. Richmond needed to get back to work. After kisses, hugs and "I love you's," they left for Reno while Kyle and I went to PACU.

We were greeted by the friendly team of nurses and Sharon, the receptionist. Kyle was tolerating the general anesthetic well enough and I was pleased with the care he was getting. With each new morning, we began our routine. I would shower, go into the kitchen and grab a quick bite while Kyle stayed in the playpen. I would also make a post-anesthesia peanut butter and jelly sandwich, grab a half-cup of coffee and get Kyle ready for the day. Then we would go to the hospital for XRT. I would grab a cup of coffee at the XRT waiting area after he was put under.

That morning I brought my camera and tripod to record Kyle being "nuked." I had already thought about the effect I wanted. As everyone tended to Kyle, I prepared to shoot the photos. The anesthesiologist appeared stunned. I looked at him and said, "If I didn't take these photos, he wouldn't have anything in his baby book." He tried to grin, but didn't say much.

One of the photos was shot through the window. It showed their movement as they tended to Kyle while he was completely still, already under a general. It was exciting to work on the series of photos. Having always been interested and active in photography, I wasn't going to let the opportunity pass. Most of the techs allowed me to take their photos, too. Documenting these events was an important part of our lives.

We met a new attending resident of anesthesiology almost daily. They were all nice and Kyle liked everyone he met, though he lacked the vocabulary to comment on their drug choices. Each doctor had his/her own preference, and I recorded each drug in my journal. Kyle was given ketamine a number of mornings. A PCP derivative, it can cause hallucinations and "ketamine dreams."

On the morning of July 30, we showed up at 8:30 a.m. for his radiation. On our way to recovery, I was pleased as Kyle began to wake up in a good mood again. We settled in at PACU so the nurses could monitor him over the coming hour. As I stood by the crib, Kyle pushed up on his arms and looked at a blank white wall.

"Hello ..." he said.

I called the nurse over.

"He's hallucinating, isn't he?" I asked.

She looked at the chart to verify ketamine as the drug of choice.

"Oh yeah, probably," she said calmly, "but it doesn't seem to bother small children, because they aren't that sure what's real and what's not."

Our son was talking to a blank wall. Great! He didn't seem upset by whatever he saw and so far I hadn't seen any evidence of "ketamine dreams." I actually found it amusing.

As I sat in recovery awaiting the customary hour, I reflected on a story Dr. Mogul had told me regarding patients and drugs. It seems Dr. Mark was in a treatment room preparing a teen-age boy for a bone marrow biopsy. The boy's father was present. He was a very conservative man, and the boy was normally very well-mannered. Dr. Mogul had given the boy versed, to help him relax and wipe out memory, and morphine to take care of the pain. As a result, the boy was awake—but not himself.

"Hey Dr. Mark," the boy said. "Come here."

"I can't," Mark said, "I'm sterile, and you're prepped."

"Hey Doc, come here." the boy repeated. So Mark leaned over the boy's face, listening carefully.

"Hey Dr. Mark," the boy said, "you're a fuckin' asshole."

As if struck by a slap, the father exclaimed, "Hey now, that's not nice." The boy looked up at his father.

"Hey," he said, "if he was sticking a needle that big in your ass, you'd think he was a fuckin' asshole, too."

Dr. Mark did his best not to laugh. He knew the father was horrified. Drugs did bizarre things to people.

THE NEXT MORNING, I woke up in a terrific mood, feeling revived and ready to go. Parking at Children's made it easier to find a space, though it was a great distance to XRT. No matter, I enjoyed the exercise. I plopped Kyle down into the stroller and took off running. As we zipped along I sang, "Nuke 'em 'til he glows, that's our motto." I thought it was a catchy little tune. Few people heard and fewer still would have appreciated my enthusiasm. Nevertheless, I sang and Kyle seemed to enjoy our daily morning jaunt.

We would arrive at XRT and one of the techs would pipe, "Hey Kyle, are you ready to go?" Kyle would smile or gurgle or say, "Hello," and they would ask him for a high-five before starting the procedures. I would have enjoyed it a lot more if that big fat door didn't slam shut. As carefree as I could be, I had a hard time each morning when the door closed and they pushed the "nuke" button.

The early morning of Aug. 1 began with a new twist. Kyle woke up screaming. Not crying or slightly upset—but flipped out. Ketamine dream? Kyle never woke up with anything other than a smile. Speaking with the Dr. that morning, I politely yet firmly suggested the anesthesiologist choose another drug. Kyle has never been given Ketamine since.

As soon as he was out of recovery, we headed home for the weekend. We arrived mid-afternoon Friday and would have all Saturday to enjoy. Sunday morning we would have to leave earlier to beat the Sunday afternoon traffic that always tied things up in the Bay area. We had a pretty good feel for the rush-hour patterns by now.

We were so battle-worn from hospital duty that it was challenging just to enjoy the time at home. Anna didn't adjust any better than the rest of us and we were all exhausted. We decided that the next weekend I would stay in Palo Alto with Kyle and try to regroup. The drive was challenging enough without all the extra stress of making a round trip.

We spent the time we had in Reno holding each other and gathering strength. We were all doing the best we could to keep a stiff upper lip. Richmond and I talked and decided he should go on his annual antelope hunt, but keep it short. Anna would be well cared for and I knew it would be good for him. I had a close friend, Joyce Wolf, who lived about two hours from Palo Alto. We had met and become friends during my roofing days in Chicago. Joyce was a redhead in her late twenties, and easy-going. She would be able to come to Palo Alto the next weekend to keep Kyle and me company. With that plan in mind, I kissed Richmond and Anna good-bye, knowing we wouldn't see them for two weeks. As we drove back to Stanford that Sunday morning, I reflected on our more carefree days.

When Anna was quite young, she, Richmond and I had camped together in the middle of nowhere. We were in our element walking in the mountains, camping under the stars and fishing in the high desert creeks. On one trip up to Summer Camp Creek in the high desert of northern Nevada, we decided the time was right to add another little bumpkin to our family. We wanted to see more children grow up. Together we could explore the world, go on adventures and, simply, enjoy life.

Never had I dreamed our distant adventures would take such a twist.

I had talked to our hospital counselor many times before. One is assigned to each family soon after diagnosis. I liked her well enough, but lately had started talking to a seminary student named Dick who came by the room on occasion. I really liked him and enjoyed our talks a great deal. Dad had given me a book, of which the title escapes me, that was his father's. It was filled with verses that could bring comfort, also.

My prayers took on a new format. I started praying for strength to enjoy the good and withstand the bad. Both qualities are necessary to keep a healthy mind amid continued difficulties. I didn't come to this practice for a few weeks—I had spent about four to six weeks not praying at all. I was so furious with God I couldn't bring myself to say a prayer. I was so angry, had I said anything to God, it would have been littered with expletives.

But my rage was short-lived, and I moved on to healthier feelings. I visited friends at Children's after Kyle's XRT for smiles or a hug.

At the front entrance of Children's Hospital are two pillars covered with hand-painted tiles. Each tile is decorated by a patient or family member while waiting for oncology appointments. The

maturity expressed by young children on some of the tiles is stag-
gering. Anna left her handprint, painted purple. There were numerous other tiles painted by children we knew. Touching Anna's tile
left me with bittersweet feelings.

Finally, the weekend arrived. I was tired and Kyle was feeling
the effects of his treatments. His spirit was good, but his energy
was marginal. He still wasn't walking, but I didn't expect him to
start romping around as we were putting him under a general
anesthetic every day!

Joyce Wolf arrived Saturday morning to keep Kyle and me
company. We were going to Montara Beach, Fisherman's Wharf,
and Moss Beach Distillery for dinner. Joyce and I had a mutual
interest in photography; we had gone on many adventures for
the sole purpose of photographing the world. After she arrived
and dropped off her things, we let Kim and Jim know when
we'd be back.

We fought our way through traffic to Fisherman's Wharf,
just barely found a parking space, and wandered around. I had
been doing a lot of that lately and was a certified wanderer.
Before long we decided to head toward the beach in search of
better photos.

Kyle was happy-go-lucky, digging his toes in the sand. Joyce and
I both enjoyed snapping photos of Kyle and the beautiful scenery.
Drained and tired as I was, the breeze from the ocean felt like a
sedative. It was nice to be away from the hospital, enjoying the
company of an old friend and laughing. We made our way back to
the car, brushed off the sand, and decided we should all get something to eat.

We arrived at the restaurant before the dinner hour and went to
a table in the bar to feast on hors d'oeuvres. Kyle, Joyce and I split
an assortment, one of which was a stuffed artichoke. It was Kyle's
favorite and the couple at the table behind found that hysterical.
The woman commented on how cute Kyle was.

"Wow, his hair is wild," she said. "Do you put mousse in it?"

"No" I replied, "It pretty much does that by itself."

I looked at Joyce and grinned. What little hair he had stood
straight up. No matter what I did to it, he looked like he had a
punk hairdo. Joyce and I enjoyed the humor of the situation.

The weekend over, it was back to XRT, in addition to Kyle's in-patient chemo. I gathered our things from Kim and Jim's. Kyle and I went to the hospital to start the day. I was battle-worn! At least we only had three more days before we could return to Reno. How bad could three days be?

I DIDN'T KNOW EXACTLY why Kyle stopped breathing and required intubation on the table, post-radiation, that day. Knowing he required a tube for breathing was upsetting. I was too engrossed in the moment to be concerned with any information other than his immediate condition. Fear reeled through my mind with as much power as the exhaustion that swept over my body.

It was awful. I was wrecked and Kyle was feeling the effects of the constant drugs. My journal notes how trying that day was:

8/13/91 Personal
Tuesday afternoon
I am almost at my wits end these days. Yesterday was tough duty. Kyle quit breathing on the table post radiation. They had to intubate and Mike (the tech) was in the room saying a Hail Mary for Kyle. They see a lot…and they were afraid for Kyle. The anesthesiologists also see a lot, and reassured me, but Kyle was in the nuke room for an extra 20 minutes before they would even move him to recovery.

We also did clinic and started chemo. Kyle threw up worse than ever. The whole thing makes me terribly afraid. His (Kyle's) last day of treatment is tomorrow and instead of being elated, I am scared to death. I was on the phone to RHB when Kyle started the "Technicolor yawn" (throwing up). I started yelling at the nurse and buzzing them and telling them I wanted Kyle's reglan and benedryl NOW!!! I didn't even have time to hang up on RHB so he was on the phone listening to the whole horrible experience.

I was up until 2 a.m. holding the basin for Kyle while he threw up . Tough duty. At one point after he threw up all over everything, I cleaned him up, the nurses changed his bed, and I changed Kyle. He then lay in my arms and on the bed. He reached over, turned my chin toward him, and gave me a kiss, as if to say, "Mom you're doing a good job." I love him dearly and he is worth every minute.

12:40 a.m. I am finally going to be able to sleep, after talking to some parents. It's hard to settle down here even when you're tired. Good Night.

Tomorrow is Kyle's...

LAST DAY OF TREATMENT ! ! ! ! !

It was the only time I had screamed at the nurses. I was frazzled—on the edge. I felt bad that Richmond had heard everything. As I threw down the phone and grabbed the buzzer for the nurse, everything went crashing off the table. I was screaming, poor Kyle was puking, and Richmond had no idea what was going on. I was almost glad he heard the chaos, because it was important for him to realize some of what we were going through. Some things are hard to understand unless you're there.

The next day, Kyle was scheduled for his last XRT treatment and MRI to measure his progress (or lack thereof), and his last scheduled dose of chemo. He would have a general anesthetic in the morning, then sedation in the afternoon for the MRI, followed by VP-16 in late afternoon or evening.

Waking up the next morning, I was thankful for a new day, our last day, and took Kyle to XRT that afternoon. It was very emotional for me. The techs had brought me smiles and casual conversation on the most frightening days of my life. They put their heart and souls behind their efforts to help cure Kyle's cancer. None of us knew if their efforts would pay off.

With the last rad administered, Kyle's XRT was complete. I wept, thanking each tech for all he and she had done. We would miss them all.

That afternoon, Kyle went into the MRI tube. His test usually took 45 minutes. I told the young woman at the desk I was going to the cafeteria to get a cup of coffee and would be right back.

When I returned to the MRI area, I saw everybody standing around a gurney. Nothing registered at first, then I realized all those people were working on Kyle. I rushed over.

I shrieked, "He's not breathing!"

"Yes," someone calmly said, "he is."

I screamed, "Not very well!"

I was hearing the same kind of slow, labored breathing I had heard from Cassie right before she died. I was falling apart and the nurse was trying to calm me by explaining what had happened and that he would be fine. The situation was under control. I sure as hell wasn't. Kyle sounded too much the way Cassie had sounded.

They had him on oxygen as Kyle was transported back to 2 North, accompanied by a half-dozen people. The walk felt especially long, with tears blinding my paces. I was overwhelmed with fear and lack of sleep. Cancer battle fatigue had me on the ropes. I was dangerously close to hysteria.

For hours, Kyle's nurse barely left his side. After Kyle's vitals stabilized, I told his nurse that a glass of liquid courage was in order before calling my husband for the second time in three days to tell him our son had "quit" breathing (or close enough to require resuscitation).

I sat in the bar at the California Cafe drinking a glass of wine and contemplating the upcoming conversation with Richmond. Thank God we were going home the next day. I returned to the hospital feeling a little more relaxed. Kyle was resting comfortably, so I sat down to call Richmond.

I dialed the phone almost hoping he wouldn't answer.

"Hello," he said.

"Hi honey," I almost whispered.

"You don't sound very good. How was your day?"

"Kyle is O.K." I paused. "But today they had to pull him out of the MRI tube. He practically quit breathing. He sounded like Cassie before she died."

"Oh my God ... how?! What happened?" he asked. "Are you sure he's OK?"

I calmly explained what I wasn't sure of myself:

"Kyle had a general in the morning for XRT. The first sedation for the MRI didn't take, so he was given another dose. He's always hard to sedate and I guess it was just too much for him. When his breathing dropped too low, they had to revive him with narcan—a drug that reverses narcotics. He's OK now...but today really stunk."

Richmond felt out of touch and too far away. I felt alone and without any reserve strength. It was awful. I didn't think I could take anymore. I was so thankful we were going home the next day, if only for a week before needing to return for the follow-up MRI.

I told Richmond that Kyle had been baptized in his hospital room. It seemed like the right thing to do. Kyle seemed so close to the abyss the whole week.

The next morning, at my request, Kyle's chemo was given as early as possible so we could go home.

We packed up our belongings and said good-bye, hoping never to stay overnight at Children's again. Kyle had been through so much and we still had to wonder if the treatments were successful.

Time would tell.

CHAPTER 17

STILL WAITING

The night Kyle and I returned home, I sat down to talk to Richmond after the kids were tucked into bed.

We had been gone for almost a month. There would be an adjustment period for all of us, especially Anna. It would be more challenging than ever because we were all incredibly tired and at wits' end.

And yet I knew I would have to call upon any reserve strength I might have to re-establish my role as mother for Anna. I didn't know if I could pull it off, but planned on doing all I could. I was full of compassion for Anna. She had been without me for a full month and was not sure how long I would stick around this time.

It was time to put our lives back together as a family. I was in tatters. I clutched at straws on a daily and even hourly basis to pull me through those difficult times. It was almost too much.

We needed Kyle's blood checked a few days after we were home. Anna, Kyle and I went to the local hospital. All was well.

A few days later, all four of us drove to Stanford. We were extremely anxious to find out what the MRI would show. We stayed at the Hyatt, since the "Willow Road Resort" was booked. Kim and Jim had guests visiting that week. After the MRI we planned to wander around the coast for the rest of the weekend.

Early that day I made some entries in my journal.

Friday 8/23/91 10:30 a.m.
We are at Stanford MRI today to finish the MRI that got canned last week.

RHB, Anna and I stayed at the Hyatt Rickies last night. The kids had a blast. Kyle must have taken 10 steps in a row at least 12 times. We were all enjoying that.

Anna is enjoying playing with Judy (the receptionist) at MRI while I am in the cafeteria and RHB waits at MRI nervously. It's nice to be able to walk away, and know someone is down there with Kyle.

There is so much to say and feel that it's hard to explain or communicate.

Candlelighters (the cancer family assistance organization) gave us $250 to assist in expenses. What a treat. That was a nice ending to a bad week that left me unbelievably frazzled. Fran (RHB's dad) even asked if they were giving me anything for stress. He gave me a few of his tranquilizers. They have helped take the edge off without a buzz at all.

I am still strong, but am not made of steel. It has helped me get back to normal.

It is good to be down here as a family.

After Kyle got out of recovery, we all loaded into the Suburban and started our drive to the coast. Judy, the receptionist in MRI, had assured me that his test would be read that afternoon. We didn't want to wait until Monday wondering what they would tell us. So with that in mind, we wandered over to a beach and played awhile. We stopped at a unique fresh-fish market right on the water and then searched out our accommodations. We found a beautiful bed and breakfast across from the water, in the little town of Pillar Point. The room was gorgeous: fireplace, big feather bed. With two small children—oops—there went the romance. The kids loved the room and the dock across the street where pelicans were diving for dinner.

Settling in, we wandered around a bit and decided to check with the hospital. Dr. Mogul wasn't in town so we tried to reach the attending physician, Dr. Russo.

She called back a short time later with the results. Richmond and I both tried to hear the information given to us from one telephone receiver.

8/23/91 5:00 p.m.
UNBELIEVABLE FEAR!!

There is something on the MRI. We will know nothing until Monday. 'It' is the size of the tumor they took out in May.

We tried to keep ourselves together for Anna and Kyle. But we knew how unforgiving cancer could be. We gathered the kids and went to dinner. The meal was a disaster. The children sensed our stress and began acting up. We left and got the kids ready for bed.

After they were asleep, we sat in the living room. I drank far more sherry than I needed. God must have given me a break because even as I went to bed I thought to myself, "Oh great, tomorrow I'll have a terrible hangover, too." But I didn't. I considered it a gift.

We ate a fabulous breakfast, but the order of the day was our rambling fears, a four-hour drive home to Reno and the waiting…

8/25/91 Sunday
We discuss death and our fears. The discussion has a brutal slap of (possible) reality that follows closely behind. I have seen too many children die in the last year and to look at them you know something is eating them alive and it's frightening, brutal, and inconceivable that we could be experiencing this—except?? Here?? We?? Are?? Or?? Are?? We??

Monday we received a call from the hospital. Nothing was certain, but the head MRI doctor thought the characteristics of the mass pointed toward a blood clot.

The catecholamine (urine) results would be helpful. That test had always picked up neuroblastoma on Kyle.

8/26/91 Personal
CELEBRATE!!

'It' is a blood clot. The head MRI lady was fairly certain that it is a blood clot due to visual differences that you only pick up after mucho experience.

Thank you God!!

Thank God we'll be home together as a family for a long time. We are elated!! Elated is gross understatement. The feelings of joy are unbelievable. Our entire family is ecstatic!!

8/27/91
*To wake up with no fear is a wonderful and unusual gift. We
are grateful and floating on air.*

A few days later we received the results of the urine test.

8/29/91
Catecholamines are normal!!!

Rejoice!!

That was fabulous news. It gave us hope that whatever "it" was,
it wasn't neuroblastoma. We knew, following Kyle's surgery, that
scar tissue was quite probable. Dr. Mogul suggested we repeat
MRI, urine and blood tests in one month along with a few other
tests. In the meantime we could stay home and try to re-learn family dynamics. A month seemed like an eternity to us at that point.
Richmond asked if I would mind if he went hunting. I loved venison and it would do him good, so I encouraged him.

Joyce, my old friend who lived near Stanford, was coming to
visit with her roommate, Mary. We would enjoy a girls' weekend
while RHB was on his hunt. Our time became filled with art projects, reading, cooking and lots of hugging. Richmond, the kids and
I were looking forward to a trip to Chicago in October.

My sister, Angie, was getting married and wanted me to be her
matron of honor. We would stay at my sister, Dawn's, house during
our trip. Angie was five years younger than I, with dark curly hair,
a gorgeous figure and mischievous smile. She could be a tough
cookie but had a heart of gold. We didn't have any mutual biological
parents but had grown up together after my Dad married her mom.

"Are you sure you want me to be the matron of honor and Anna
to be the flower girl?" I asked Angie. "You know we might have to
bail out on you, and you'll only have half a wedding party."

"That's the way I want it," she replied. "If you can't be there, it
will all work out."

Wish Upon A Star, an organization that grants wishes to children
with life-threatening illnesses, offered to buy our plane tickets to
Chicago and give us some spending money. They were funded
through the California Highway Patrol. We were very thankful
since we couldn't afford the expense of the trip at that time.

As our upcoming trip to Stanford crept closer, I knew I couldn't make it alone with Kyle. Richmond had to be by my side. If we got bad news again, taking it alone would be more than I could handle. I had taken too many bad blows by myself, through no fault of Richmond.

Our fourth wedding anniversary was also the day of Kyle's next MRI and we wanted to be together, no matter what we were doing. We rented a nice hotel room—very romantic—oops! There were those two kids again. Nevertheless, we needed somewhere to stay. A day or two later, the "Willow Road Resort" would be available.

Depending on the MRI, Kyle's tests could last many days. Richmond would meet us at the Hyatt the afternoon after the MRI so we could hear the news together. He would return to Reno shortly thereafter to keep pace with his work while Anna, Kyle and I stayed for the remainder of the tests. Richmond arrived at the hotel and we looked over the room service menu as we waited for Dr. Mark to call with the results. Richmond brought a bottle of wine, popped the cork and poured us each a glass. We ordered up some goodies for everyone to enjoy and toasted to our love. We enjoyed the evening and the kids. Try as they did to stay awake, they were sound asleep before long.

Late that evening, the phone rang. Dr. Mark was on the line. Once again, Richmond and I craned our ears to hear. We could barely make our Mark's voice on the phone and hoped we had misunderstood. I took the receiver and asked him to repeat.

Unfortunately, it was what we thought we'd heard. The previously detected mass was 2 centimeters larger. There also was something in one of Kyle's lymph nodes in the pelvic region.

Richmond and I hardly knew what to say. We decided I would stay at Stanford with Anna and Kyle while the upcoming tests were completed. Mark said there would be a few days of testing and a biopsy would be scheduled within the week. We would still go to Chicago for Angie's and wedding. Until then, Richmond would be running his business.

The next morning, Anna, Kyle and I kissed Richmond good-bye and went to the hospital for tests. By then, Kyle had already had a number of bone scans. The bone scan would show cancer if it moved into Kyle's bones. If it had, the prognosis would not be good. His chances of recovery would be very slim and we weren't prepared to cross that bridge. Sitting in the room waiting was almost unbearable. Anna was always good and the hospital personnel usually seemed to come up with something to entertain her. My patience was a limited resource and I really appreciated their help.

> **9/29/91 Personal**
> *I am frazzled having both kids down here for all these tests, but readjusting would be out of the question (with Anna and I apart again) considering the upcoming trip to Chicago.*
>
> *Kim and I had a real nice talk tonight. We discussed anti-anxiety drugs, and my prescription and she reassured me after I asked her for advice. We also discussed oncology and how far in her opinion some of the doctors will go to "save" a patient. She said that by tomorrow we might at least know whether its a tumor or not—what kind—maybe 3-5 days.*
>
> *I need my sleep. Tomorrow is clinic, bone marrow, needle biopsy and 3:00 p.m. audiology. Kyle and Anna are both such great kids, that though part of me has addressed this as a clinical matter, my emotional side is heavy into denial. I am not ready to look at the possibility of losing Kyle. God help us with the upcoming events.*
>
> *RHB—I love you and miss you. You are the best. Good night.*

THE NEXT MORNING, WE went in for Kyle's needle biopsy. We were at Day Hospital and Kyle was hooked up to saline before the sedation was to be administered. Dr. Mogul and Dr. Hartman, and a radiologist came into the room.

"Kyle doesn't need a needle biopsy," they said.

I immediately flared. "You will do a biopsy and today!"

"The mass has characteristics of scar tissue," Dr. Mark said calmly. "If Dr. Hartman did a needle biopsy, there is always the chance that the biopsy would be inconclusive."

"So are we just supposed to wait another month to see what 'it' does?!"

Dr. Hartman, also a quieting force, replied, "A needle biopsy is invasive and if part of the mass was neuroblastoma and part of it wasn't, we might only get samples from the benign mass, leaving us with no more information than we had before. The catecholamines (urine test) will give us some information and we can do another MRI in a month." ·

"Great!" I replied, "So we're just supposed to wait?!"

"Call Richmond and see what he says," Dr. Mogul said. "We don't recommend it at this point."

Well, I knew what Nature Boy would say. He would think it was great—no invasive tests! I was forced to consider that waiting was the best choice. Patience wasn't my high suit. I wanted to know what "it" was and I really wanted to know immediately.

"Wait another month?" I said out loud. Melissa, Kyle's nurse, said, "Who is going to help mom survive the month?" I knew she was talking about sedatives; we knew each other quite well. I replied, "Don't worry, I've already got that covered."

So the decision was made to wait. Bone marrow was clear, bone scan clear, and, hopefully, the urine test would be clear. There was nothing to do but wait. For the time being, stress relief was the order of business. Anna, Kyle and the testing were wearing me out.

We cooked very little and ate out a lot. Max's Opera Cafe was one of our favorites. The food was great, the atmosphere fun, and it was in the neighborhood.

In a few days, Wish Upon A Star would send us on a vacation to Chicago for Angie's wedding. Kyle would be able to spend time with many of his family members whom he had not even met. Our Stanford counselor had "suggested" we take a trip.

After all, things weren't looking that good.

Then you
go home

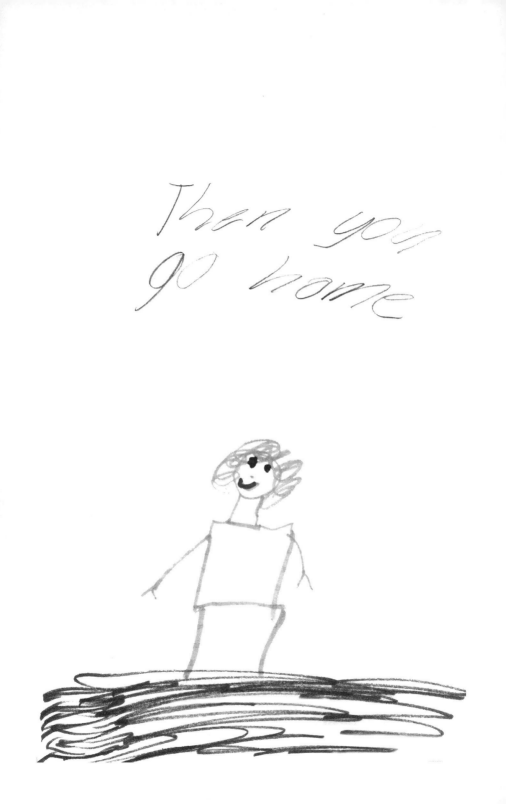

CHAPTER 18

FALL AND CHRISTMAS

We flew to Chicago on what was the bumpiest flight I had ever been on. Anna laughed her head off and Richmond, in true Nevada fashion, was heard saying, "Let's rodeo!" Kyle was pretty unaffected and myself—I kept hoping my stomach would hold up so I could stave off the "Technicolor yawn."

We enjoyed the wedding—Anna and I participating—the days visiting family, and a fun evening to Greek Town with Robin and her husband, Jay. Kyle and Anna played with their cousins on the front lawn, laughing and running back and forth as I shot pictures.

We did our best to put all the question marks in the backs of our minds during our trip, knowing that in a few more weeks there would be another MRI. The kids had a great time with their cousins, Kelly and Erin, and we relished the much-needed rest.

When we returned to Reno we went on with our daily lives. I watched as Richmond did a commendable job and his business continued to grow. Calling on clients and courting jobs must have been very difficult for him when our son was so sick. Anna and Kyle had fun together and I loved watching them interact.

Nervously waiting for the results of the catecholamines (urine test) made it difficult for me to keep focused on how fortunate we were to be together. Many times each day while watching the children, I would thank God for giving us this time. Every night at dinner and bed, Anna would pray, "Dear God, please make Kyle all better."

On Oct. 13, Mark Mogul called. Kyle's catecholamines were clear. Thank God!!

It was a very good sign, yet Richmond and I still worried something was growing inside our son. Still, the catecholamines were a big milestone since they had been an accurate marker for Kyle's cancer.

We always called family as soon as we received news, since everyone anxiously awaited the results. The good news always made me cry, and the change in my voice always made the receiver of the call very nervous. Words could never sum up the relief felt by everyone in our family.

As our scheduled MRI on Oct. 28 approached, we could cut the tension with a knife. Richmond and I found ourselves incredibly edgy. I kept in touch with the Lupros and our other hospital friends. Kendra continued to do well and her spirit was my inspiration. I reflected on how lucky I felt. Our son was still alive and full of happiness.

10/23/91 Personal

Kyle is 17 months old today. 14 months of fear, terror, loss of friends and my own self that has been partially replaced by someone less optimistic—and lots of learning. We have learned a lot about courage and have found out what we're made of. We are a tougher lot for it—that much is for sure.

I was trying to think of all the kids that died that I knew (though some not very well) from the hospital.

1. *Hannah*

2. *Janet*

3. *Chris Benninghoff*

4. *Cassie Lupro*

5. *J.P.*

6. *Pat Lindemann*

7. *Thomas*

8. *Brent*

9. *Avalia*

10. *Sherry*

I fear there are already those I've forgotten. It is a hazard of the "job." Memory loss—it's for health's sake.

There had been so many children—many tears. I was afraid that we were waiting our turn in line. Whenever I had that thought, I pushed it back and pushed optimism forward.

Richmond and I decided for MRIs Kyle would go under a general anesthetic instead of sedation. We felt the general was a much more exact science and with sedation, he occasionally had to be sedated twice. It seemed full of question marks and the anesthetic was always on target. We also decided Kyle and I would go down to Stanford by ourselves since we knew there was a growing mass.

On Oct. 27, Kyle and I enjoyed another beautiful drive over the pass, through the Sacramento Valley and across the Bay Bridge.

10/28/91 Medical
Clinic—Height 76cm, Weight 10.2 kg MRI at 1:30ish.
General Anesthesia

*Atropine

*Penethol

*Halothane

*Propofol

Intubate (Tube down throat to keep airway open) after Halothane.

Blood work came back—Alk Phos (Alkaline Phosphatase) was high (over 6,000—normal tops at 300). Dr. Mogul orders an emergency bone scan and skeletal survey. 10/29 @ 10:00 a.m.

11:15 a.m., MRI—NO CHANGE THANK GOD!

10/29/91 Personal
Kyle and I are waiting at Nuke med. for a Bone Scan. His Alk Phos was high (blood work) and that's a bone flag. Could be awful—could be nothing. The MRI was the same as last month. I am not (greatly) worried. We are also getting a full skeletal survey today.

Home tomorrow?!

Bone dye injection at 11:00 a.m. Skeletal survey at 1:45 p.m. Bone scan at 3:00 p.m. 1 dose of chloral hydrate to sleep. All (both tests) CLEAR!!

Late that evening I continued my journal entries.

Thank God! There is no explanation for the 6,000+ Alk Phos. For a few minutes I had the fear cross over me that this was going to be it, and it was in his bones. We are all tired AGAIN!—and ready for a reprieve.

Blood work in a month +/- and Hickman removal will be scheduled if/when the catecholamines come back clear.

This is exhausting work. Kyle is most definitely worth it.

Rest will come easy tonight. I have been thankful to have Kim and Jim for friends. They are wonderful people. They have been so patient with me.

I used to kid the doctors, nurses and other caregivers saying, "You guys just won't let us leave without scaring us." It seemed to me, no matter what the intended schedule was, we were always compelled to stay longer for some reason. Even at that point, I packed for a week every time we went down because I never knew when we would be able to leave.

Home we went to await catecholamine results. I always made Dr. Mark promise he would call us the second (not minute or hour or day) he got the results.

11/11/91
CELEBRATE!!

Catecholamines are NORMAL!! What an overwhelming gift. We will schedule to have his Hickman removed. We will also have Kyle tested to check his ability to handle vaccines.

Kyle never got all of his baby shots. Many vaccines are live viruses, which is a big no-no for cancer patients. They could get the disease, since their immune systems were compromised. Kyle was way behind in his immunization schedule and we wanted to ensure that his body could accept the vaccines.

The holidays approached and we were busy shopping for turkeys and other items. Some days were light-hearted, others heavy. At Saint Mary's we had Kyle's blood drawn to see how his counts were recovering. They were great.

The holiday activities continued with our annual visit to Santa. It just so happened a Reno news station was filming the children and their requests. As our turn came, Anna and Kyle both climbed in Santa's lap.

Santa said, "Ho, ho, ho, Merry Christmas. Have you been good girls and boys?" Kyle, only 18 months, didn't reply but sat smiling. As the camera zoomed in, Anna replied, "Yes." Santa asked, "What do you want for Christmas?" Anna looked up into Santa's eyes and replied, "I want there to be no more cancer in my family. I want my brother to be all better."

Needless to say, this sound bite made the 5 o'clock news. Anna's wish was so sweet and her only request. I think Santa was blown away by this 3-year-old's Christmas wish, as I imagine many viewers were.

With the possibility of the Hickman being removed, we had to schedule a surgery at Stanford a few days after the MRI—providing the MRI was still looking good. I wanted the Hickman out by Christmas. That was at the top of my Christmas list. I also thought it would be nice if we could schedule surgery around the Doobie Brothers concert. For 17 years, the band had played each Christmas in the hospital cafeteria for the children. It would be a very special concert—and maybe our last. And so the schedule went: clinic and MRI on the 16th, Doobie Brothers on the 18th and Hickman removal (hopefully) on the 19th. Home for Christmas!

As our appointment and Christmas came closer, I had to make sure I had all my ducks in a row. All the presents were bought and wrapped. I was as prepared as possible and hoping they would actually let us leave the hospital without scares or delays. My sister, Angie, was going to accompany us down to Children's for tests, the Doobies concert and (hopefully) the Hickman removal.

We planned on dragging Kyle around to restaurants and maybe the local brewery. We were going to have some fun no matter what. I needed a list of supplies if Kyle continued to have a Hickman. One of the items was a hypodermic needle box. We had our own box just like the hospitals have mounted on walls. Ours was full of all the needles we had used over the seven-month period. I had special plans for that needle box. If our surgery to remove the Hickman, scheduled with Dr. Hartman, was completed, he would get a surprise.

Angie, Kyle and I met Richmond and Anna at a friend's Christmas party in Napa. We really enjoyed ourselves, but knew at the end of the day we were going to Stanford again while Richmond and Anna were returning home. When it was time to go, Richmond and I walked down the long driveway to be alone. Angie had the kids, while Richmond and I hugged and said good-bye. We were battle-worn and hopeful that the MRI results would be in Kyle's favor.

Angie and I put Kyle in his car seat. "Hey, Kyle," I said. "Let's go see our friends at the hospital!" He smiled and uttered baby gurgles of one kind or another and we were on our way to the "Willow Road Resort."

Early the next morning we went to the hospital. I wanted to introduce Angie to our friends. She wanted to see for herself what we had been doing the past 16 months. First we went to the clinic, which was full of a number of bald chemo kids, and then for the MRI.

After Kyle's tests, we went up to 2 North to see if anyone we knew was there. Kendra wasn't in and the board had only unfamiliar names. We couldn't get MRI results until later that day. We stopped and visited the nurses, who were always thrilled to see Kyle. He loved all the hugs he got.

I had spent so much time at Children's Hospital that upon returning there were many friends to visit. Later that day, the MRI results came in. The mass had shrunk! Tumors didn't shrink, cancer didn't shrink—scar tissue did!

The nationwide Kyle alert hit the phone lines with joyful exclamation heard on all fronts. Kyle would be tubeless for Christmas!

We were overjoyed and knew that we had a chance—maybe he would never have cancer again. We could hope and we already prayed. Surgery was on the 19th and I wouldn't have to do Hickman care, heparin locks, or care if the area of his shirt that was over his Hickman got soaked in front from baby drool.

Angie, Kyle and I went out and celebrated, had a great dinner and brought wine back to Kim and Jim's. Richmond and I had grown accustomed to taking really good or bad news over the phone. He celebrated on his end and we on ours. It was a great ending to a long day.

The next day we took our time. Waking up knowing the good news continued was a terrific feeling. We went to the Doobie Brothers concert in the hospital cafeteria. It was a very special day.

The Doobies opened with, "Listen to the Music." There is a line in that song about making people smile—they know how to do that. After watching a concert with onlookers who had a multitude of diseases (many life-threatening) and an array of IV poles, Angie had a new view on life. The smiling faces surrounded by adversity were inspiring. There wasn't a dry eye when the Doobies sang, "Silent Night." I still get tears in my eyes when I hear some of their songs on the radio.

The next morning we were at the hospital bright and early for Kyle's general anesthetic and the Hickman removal by Dr. Hartman.

The resident walked in the room. "Hello," she said. "I'm the resident anesthesiologist and Kyle will be going in soon. Do you have any questions?"

"I would like him to have halothane, maybe a little versed," I replied. "No propofol, it makes him really cranky."

She looked surprised. "Are you an anesthesiologist?"

"No, I'm just a participating parent."

After the Hickman removal, Dr. Hartman came out and let us know that everything had gone well. Hickman removal is relatively simple, so I wasn't worried. I did have something I wanted to give the doctor.

"Can you sit down for a minute?" I asked, patting the seat next to me. "This isn't your typical Christmas present, but it's appropriate."

He looked at me sideways with a slight grin.

"You were the first one to say 'neuroblastoma' and you are taking out his last Hickman," I continued.

He tore open the paper and chuckled at the box full of needles as Sharon, the receptionist at PACU, took our picture. We had to return the needle box to the hospital anyway for disposal and I thought this was a humorous way to do it.

Dr. Hartman deserved the laugh he got out of it. He was a great guy who always stopped to answer a question or just say, "Hi." I could always count on a smile from him, too. He and Schocat were a terrific surgical team with good bedside manners; but we hoped we would never have to see them again.

Angie and I took Kyle, our Tubeless Wonder, to the car for our ride home. Instead of a tube, there was only a Band-Aid. That was so great, and the timing for Christmas even better.

12/20/91 Personal
We are home and Hickmanless. It really hasn't sunk in. I have spent today crying, off and on, mostly due to relief that we are getting a reprieve.

Johnny Stevens (a little boy with neuroblastoma) is dying— maybe at this moment. The cancer is actually breaking his bones. He is on a lot of morphine. Quite sad and unreal what cancer can do. They had Christmas a week ago.

Kim Stevens (Johnny's Mom) said, 'Never drop your guard. As soon as we did he relapsed.' I know intellectually it doesn't work that way but emotionally we feel we will always be 'cautiously optimistic.'

We pray for continued strength. I feel weaker now than a week ago in certain ways. It's such a relief that the dam has to break just for release.

We have some hope now, and we will keep enjoying each day we have together as a family.

We enjoyed the holidays that year, finding the simplest things most inspiring. Hospital life was no longer the front-runner. We weren't due back for three months. It almost seemed too long, and initially made me very nervous. So much could grow in that period.

We were learning to live without the hospital or appointments looming over our heads. The fear was still present, but receded every day.

We decided against a Christmas letter that year, deciding instead to send a New Year's letter with a family photo taken at Montara Beach in August.

IT IS A NEW YEAR!

The beach is a special place, just over the hill from Stanford. We enjoy coming here. I feel we have gathered some strength and insight here. I remember as a child being taught never to turn my back on the ocean, for you never know when a big wave might sweep you out to sea... I found myself teaching Anna this lesson the day we took this picture.

We turned our backs to cancer once, but never again. A wary eye shall forever be with us now. When Kyle relapsed in May, a harsh and bitter wave of reality slammed into us, threw us, tumbled and bashed us with a crushing weight, made us gasp for breath and flung us onto the sand, wasted, wondering, what happened? We wrote you in April and proclaimed Kyle "Cancer Free." This was unfortunately premature. May 20th the doctors at Stanford found that a tumor had reoccurred in his pelvis where the original tumor was. It is fortunate that we had a few months between February and May to regain some strength and courage for what lay ahead.

May 29th Kyle underwent another major surgery in which a second tumor was removed. Ten days after surgery Kyle was put through four rounds of intense chemotherapy concurrent with a month of radiation during which time, each day, he was put under general anesthetic to ensure that he would not move while being irradiated by an electron beam. His treatments were completed August 15th. It was a summer of great fears and anxieties. Since August, Kyle has had four Magnetic Resonance Image tests plus numerous other tests. December 16th we received the best Christmas gift possible as Kyle had a checkup and the doctor's were very optimistic saying everything looked good and they don't want to see us until March 9th for his next checkup. We are told that we need to get five years of checkups behind us now before we can consider neuroblastoma gone from our lives ...

It is such a wonderful gift having our family together again after so much separation through the past sixteen months. Donna calculates that she and Kyle were away from home six and a half months during the past period. Watching Kyle and Anna play together is a true joy. We are incredibly lucky to have Kyle after all that has transpired. He is so happy and full of the dickens, you would never believe he has had to endure all of this. Anna continues to blossom. Her love of life, her brother and family is astounding considering how her little life has been tossed and tumbled about this past sixteen months. Her command of the English language is such fun to hear, quite impressive actually, and supremely entertaining. Her observation of a World Series outfielder catching a fly ball was a unique assessment, "Daddy, he made a basket in his mitten." Well, basketball, baseball, who cares? They're all fun sports! We have a wonderful time together.

We grew our best crop of garlic (thus far) this summer, 10-15 lbs. The problem is that we already ate it all. Baked garlic can really blow through a good stash of bulbs! YUM. Well, you see our copious garlic consumption can be explained. In days of old, the sages, shamans, and healers knew that garlic possessed magic powers against evil. There are numerous legends attributing garlic with great powers to increase strength, speed and endurance. The Egyptian slaves ate garlic as they built the pyramids, and the Romans took it to strengthen them in battle. Need we say more...?

Gardening, working around the home front and cooking delicious meals of wild game, fish and home grown vegetables have taken on special meaning for Donna and I this year. The grounding and healing energy derived from these pursuits have been so welcomed and needed.

This year running the landscape business was a greater challenge that ever before. Gee, I can't imagine why?!!! But, amidst it all, the business grew and was filled with many exciting, challenging and rewarding projects. There were a couple of fine hunts with bow and arrow for deer and antelope this fall. A fine four-point mule deer was a beautiful gift from the mountains. The venison has been exceptional. The vastness and beauty of Nevada's high desert country continue to replenish my spirit.

Our hearts, souls and spirits have also been continuously nourished and blessed by your kind words, deeds and prayers. Our families have gone beyond the call of duty. The doctors and staff at Stanford have done a tremendous job. All this love and compassion has made our year an easier trial.

For this, we are forever grateful and give thanks. Here's to a Healthy, Happy New Year!

All our love to you,

Richmond, Donna, Anna and Kyle

CHAPTER 19

KENDRA

As the days and weeks passed, we were adjusting to normal life. It was all so easy. When I heard people bitch about their "problems," I just grinned and thought back on our not-so-distant problems. Big difference. Our perspective was on a completely different plane, and our lives were beginning to feel grounded.

We still knew that Kyle was a gift (as was Anna), but that we might not have a whole lot of time with him. Battling cancer is not an exact science. We were all in great need of a vacation after our trip "to hell and back." I started researching getaways where we could all have a good time.

A vacation before his next MRI sounded good. Somewhere warm, tropical, relaxing. *Money* you say? *Visa* I said!

As my sister, Dawn, said, "Let's spend future money." I booked a trip for Anna, Kyle, Richmond and me to Club Med Ixtapa. It was a family resort in Mexico with stuff for the kids to do, leaving the parents with free time. The trip sounded perfect and if Kyle's next MRI wasn't up to par—well, anyway, we deserved it. We scheduled the trip for the week before our visit to Stanford. We would go directly from the beach to the hospital, which would eliminate a lot of the pre-appointment stress.

We also discussed having another baby. Three would be a great number; one was never a choice for me. Richmond wanted us to research the genetic possibility of neuroblastoma occurring again in our lives. I called a genetic counselor at Stanford, and mailed her all the information she requested. We would meet with her on March 9, before we went to the clinic. As our trip and next MRI approached, I logged an entry in my journal:

2/22/92
*Last night I dreamt that after a routine pap exam, I was told
I had tumors. Do you suppose I am worried about Kyle's
upcoming MRI?!? (2 weeks from now) I feel myself squashing
the fears and concentrating on our upcoming trip to Mexico
(2/28-3/7) We are greatly looking forward to it. I have seen
myself continually scream at Anna and Kyle the week prior
to MRI—often unnecessarily and followed by apologies by
myself to Anna or Kyle, or Richmond. Last MRI I even dreamt
I had cancer and decided to kill myself because I didn't think
Richmond would be able to cope with the kids, and a chemo
series for me. It wasn't that I was depressed, thus offing
myself. It was much more like I just thought it was the practical thing to do. I suppose some of this is the old 'if it could
be me and not you Kyle, I'd do it' I don't know if I would or
not—I don't know if I'm that strong, and I also know there's
no choice anyway, so thinking that way is a waste of time.*

As it turned out, we were too busy playing in the sand, eating
like royalty and drinking tropical drinks to even think about
Stanford—or at least, not much. We left the beach and boarded a
plane. The next morning we went to the hospital for Kyle's scheduled appointments. We were well rested and anxiously awaited
the upcoming test. We arrived at the clinic first.

The blood counts were good, the MRI showed the mass had
shrunk again, and the catecholamines were clear!

Another clean appointment under our belt felt good. We
remained cautiously optimistic. I continued to keep in touch with
our hospital friends. The Lupros were doing as well as could be
expected and other friends were hanging in there. Kendra was
still doing well. I always enjoyed talking to her mom and dad,
Sharon and David.

Our next appointment at Stanford was going to be our first
stop on a trip to my grandfather's 98th birthday party. It was in
June and my mom was flying to Reno. Then she, Anna, Kyle and I
were going on a 1,500-mile adventure with the children. I couldn't
have driven it alone and our bills required Richmond to keep his
nose to the grindstone. As before, we felt a great amount of pre-
checkup stress.

THE VERY FIRST DAY of clinic I heard a boy talking about
when his parents found out he had cancer.

"They were really bummed," he said.

That was Ozzie, and though I didn't get to know him well, news from Dr. Mogul about his death brought sadness to my heart. He had never known he had given me strength at a critical time in my life. When I heard him speak casually about his disease and day of diagnosis, he got my attention. The strength he showed was impressive.

We all tried to keep the stress level down as our upcoming checkup and big adventure to papa's birthday party approached. And there was another development. We were expecting a baby. I was only a few weeks along, at which point I was tired and cranky anyway. Stanford stress just multiplied my crankiness.

Richmond kissed us good-bye and wished us luck on the big adventure. Upon arrival at Stanford, all that Kyle needed was clinic, blood and urine tests.

We checked in and waited our turn. Kyle didn't cry during the blood draw. He even thanked the phlebotomist! His pain threshold was higher than mine—that was for sure.

While talking to Dr. Mogul during Kyle's checkup, I asked if he and Robin had stopped at any really great spots on the coast. We were only planning on driving four hours or so a day, for all of our sakes. Any recommendations would be appreciated. He suggested Point Lobos, a nature reserve and park. There would be seals and many other ocean animals. The kids would love it.

I was psyched—but there was bad news. Kendra Green had relapsed. They would start a bone-marrow transplant the next day. I prayed: God, please don't let Kendra die.

This news was a terrible blow. Kendra was such a great girl and we had always held onto the fact that she was doing well. She had a completely different disease, but in the back of my mind if she was doing well—we could, too. In a way, she symbolized my hope.

I called my sister, who had met Kendra the very first night when Kendra talked to us about how chemo was no big deal. Dawn also was devastated. I sat down and just cried.

We continued on our trip, but I thought about Kendra many times a day. She would be getting a bone-marrow transplant where they used her own marrow. Since her bones were still "clean," they had harvested her marrow so they could give her "big guns" chemo. Then they could inject the marrow in the hopes that it would produce healthy cells, thus ridding her body of cancer. She would be in a double-door isolation room to maintain a germ-free environment for about two months. Then time would tell.

It was fun seeing family and my healthy 98-year-old grandfather at his birthday party. Anna and Kyle played in the swimming pool and drove the golf cart around the mobile home park. With two small children it wasn't very relaxing, but we still had fun. I tried to concentrate on enjoying the trip. Without our results, and hearing Kendra's news, made it more difficult.

One night when Mom, Anna, Kyle and I were still on our trip, I had a dream. It was a long, detailed dream in which Mark Mogul told us the catecholamine results were "slightly elevated." More tests would be done sooner and if Kyle had relapsed, we would be in for a bone-marrow transplant.

I bolted up in bed sweating and went to Kyle's bed to put my hands on him. I was mortified and couldn't shake the dream. It took me about an hour-and-a-half before I could think of anything else. It had been so real.

The next day, we arrived home. Richmond had missed us a great deal. It was good to be back. We replayed various tales of our adventures and spent time regrouping from our long drive. We still hadn't heard from Dr. Mogul about Kyle's urine test.

Late Saturday we received a phone call. I recorded it in my journal:

> **6/20/92**
> *Our cat # (catecholamine) is up. Bad news. MRI and next urine test moved up two months. Not the news we wanted.*
>
> *Mogul called us immediately upon his return from vacation. 10:00 p.m. Saturday night. That's a wonderful doctor. If the tumor is back, we will have to do another surgery followed by a bone marrow transplant (B.M.T.) It would be autologous (Kyle's own bone marrow) and the recovery time is supposed to be much quicker. So, once again we are in limbo. We will know more 7/6 when Kyle's next MRI is. I can't believe we are even having to think about B.M.T. we will make it through whatever is ahead. We feel strong.*

The phone call was so bizarre because it was ominously close to my dream. Dr. Mogul repeated verbatim, "The catecholamines are slightly elevated." We discussed the "what ifs," because I wanted to know what we might be up against. I was an optimist, but I also liked to be prepared and knew how quickly life could change when cancer rounded the bend. I asked him various questions about bone-marrow transplants. He gave me some stats on recovery times, all the while stressing that there might not be any problem at all.

"Let's do an MRI," Dr. Mark said, "repeat the urine test and take it from there."

I attempted in the next few weeks to complete any and all tasks that would make life easier on Richmond and Anna as well as family members who helped with Anna's care. Mom was flying home to Dallas. I bought a three-month supply of drinks, paper goods, dog food, etc. I mentally went down the checklist and made a serious effort to be as prepared as possible. Best-case scenario— our garage was full of things we would use, anyway. Worst-case scenario—we were as prepared as possible and could do the job of helping Kyle through a bone-marrow transplant.

Kyle's MRI was scheduled for July 6.

7/6/92 Personal
Today is the day. Hopefully we will hear good news, and have some answers.

We are all petrified, and the thought of getting bad news again is almost too much.

Part of me is convinced we will be down here all summer (as if that would help if we got bad news anyway). But the brain works in funny ways. We visited Kendra and her ANC is 6000 (boosted by drug helpers). She will be out as soon as her infection goes away. She is only twenty-one days post BMT. She is sick of being in the same room every moment of every day, but otherwise she seems to be doing well. Of course she looks like hell if you compare to the real world, but that's not a good comparison right now.

7/6/92 Medical
Height—85cm; Weight—12.2 kg

MRI at 12:30 p.m.

Anesth.   *Halothane
*   *N20*
*   *Propofol*

Kyle's asleep at 1:00 p.m.

4:30 p.m. Mogul says MRI is CLEAR

Thank God! The huge mass of fear is gone and replaced by
curiosity for the post-cat (catecholamine) results. So far so
good! Life goes on!

Our other thoughts were regarding the immunization schedule
to complete Kyle's baby shots. Dr. Mogul talked to one of the
immune specialists, who said Kyle might not be able to finish his
baby shots until pre-kindergarten.Tests could be done to find out,
but it would take quite awhile for Kyle's system to return to normal. Normal? I could hardly remember what normal was! What
really amazed me was that they could "poison" his body so much
that he couldn't even get most baby shots—yet it didn't kill him.
Astounding, in my opinion.

On July 16, Dr. Mogul called. The "cats"—catecholamines—
were back, and they were perfect! We were elated. Clear cats and
a beautiful MRI.We had jumped another hurdle and landed on the
side of normal life. We spent the rest of the summer watching the
weeds take over our garden.We had been too engulfed in fear earlier
in the summer when the weeds first appeared and they had taken
over our normally well-cared-for garden.

Early that fall, we took Kyle on his first camping trip.
Richmond, Anna, Kyle and I went up to the high northern Nevada
desert for a long weekend. We saw antelope and wild horses,
hiked, and fully enjoyed one of life's pleasures—the big beautiful
mountains of Nevada.

OUR APPOINTMENTS WERE THREE months apart.The upcoming set of tests included audio testing to see how much hearing
loss Kyle had incurred from the cisplatin chemo. He seemed to us
to hear OK, and we really didn't expect a problem. (Where had I
heard that before?)

Kyle and I went to Stanford as Richmond worked and Anna
stayed with Dad and Leigh.

10/5/92 9:00 a.m.—Hearing test
10:00 a.m.—Cats and clinic

Height—85cm; Weight—12.7 kg (28 1b.)

Hearing test practically complete. Return tomorrow to finish.
Currently called a 'significant' hearing loss. Will have trouble
with letters F,S,K,TH. Doesn't hear hissy, airy kind of sounds.

*Will need 2 hearing aids. Critical language development
years are 0-3 yrs.*

*Even with aids, background noise will make it difficult for
him to hear properly.*

Kyle sat on my lap in a sound-proof room during his audiology
test. They played different noises on both sides on the room,
switching off to see which ear could hear which sounds. It was
never clearer to me than when he was on my lap that morning. I
could hear sounds clearly and Kyle heard nothing. It made me cry,
even though I knew we were incredibly lucky. Richmond could
hardly believe it as Kyle seemed to hear well enough.

As it turned out, for a full year he hadn't been albe to hear well
at all, though some days in our lives were so loud that I honestly
thought it would be a benefit to be partially deaf.

We got clear catecholamines again and made another hurdle.
We were due back in three months for our next appointment.

The hearing-aid issue was going to require some research and
reality checks. It made us angry that Kyle had already gone
through so much, and now needed the devices. Richmond wasn't
convinced there was a problem. I told him, "The only way you will
see and understand is to hold Kyle on your lap during a test."

We called the audiologist recommended in our area, one Mike
LeMay. We met him and thought he was terrific. Richmond went
along and was able to experience first-hand what I had been trying to explain. He came out of the room with tears in his eyes.

The hearing aids were ordered at $600 apiece. Ouch! I could
just see Kyle feeding one of those to the dogs. Thank goodness
they were insurable.

The day Mike LeMay was ready to fit Kyle with the aids, we didn't
know what to expect. Kyle sat in a chair as Mike put the first
device in.

Mike said into the ear, "Hi, Kyle, how are you doing?" Kyle's face
lit up in awe as he turned and looked at Mike. He immediately
pointed to his other ear as if to say, "Where's the other one?" It was
beautiful to see Kyle's transformation over the next few weeks.
His speech improved dramatically and the little boy "who wasn't
listening very well" showed great improvement in his behavior.

It was a lot easier to do what I asked since he could finally hear what was being said. We were thankful that Stanford had sent a yearly reminder card. The damage from cisplatin is usually complete a year post-treatment. Working with Mike LeMay was a joy. Never had a 2-year-old sat as well for all the tests or while Mike made the molds that fit inside Kyle's ears.

The fall continued, with me getting plumper by the week. Our next scheduled appointment was about three weeks before I was due to deliver. Traveling far from home at that late date was not an option. We decided when we should travel and called Dr. Mark. He scheduled us for March 8. While waiting for Kyle's appointment, we enjoyed the holiday's and the new year—1993—began.

On Jan. 20, Haley Marie Breen was born, weighing in at 7 lbs., 7 oz. She was a beautiful baby girl and we all enjoyed the new dynamics of a family of five.

I continued to keep in touch with our hospital friends. Many had lost a child to cancer. The beginning of February, I called Kendra's parents, Sharon and David. Her relapse continued.

> **2/4/93**
> *Kendra relapsed. The news for Kendra is not good. Rhabdo (rabdomyosarcoma) is in her foot now, which post B.M.T.(Bone Marrow Transplant) is a sign that it will be everywhere, and there is nothing they can do. I've talked to both Sharon and Kendra. They sound good. They found out around Thanksgiving. Kendra is busy fitting as much of life in as possible. She bought a new jeep, ski vacations, Mexico, moving out on her own with her boyfriend (who was with her through it all) to Colorado. She'll be 18 in May. It will probably be her last birthday. Kendra is one incredible young lady.*

At that point in our lives, we felt very lucky that Kyle's good health continued. Kendra's fall in health brought a great deal of sadness. She had been at Stanford Children's Hospital our first night, and talking to her had brought me strength. Before she walked into our room that night a few years before, I was having serious doubts about my coping abilities. After I heard Kendra's rendition of chemo I felt like I could survive the situation. She had given me hope—an immeasurable gift. My heart ached for her and her family about her imminent death.

5/8/93
*Today is Kendra's 18th Birthday (and Mother's Day). I talked
to Sharon a week ago, and the Rhabdo (rabdomyosarcoma)
is everywhere. Kendra and Tom (her boy friend of 3+ years)
moved to Fort Collins, CO. She is enjoying being on her own.
"Tom and I go to the grocery store and we don't have to buy
anything we don't like. It's great! And...we both like Honey
Nut Cheerios." That Tom must be an incredible young man.*

*We are freaking out as we have another appointment and it
is the same scenario as when he relapsed 2 years ago.
Intellectually no comparison—emotionally—heaps.*

We pray for Kendra and her family for strength and courage.

Kyle and I continued to travel to Stanford by ourselves with
Anna often opting to join us despite the long drive. Haley also
joined the traveling group as the baby in tow. By that time MRIs
weren't standard procedure and the urine results didn't come in for
about 10 days. The blood work wasn't our most important test, so I
was in little danger of having to take bad news by myself.
Whenever we went to the hospital we visited our friends, which
Anna, Kyle and I all enjoyed very much. There were many wonderful
people at Stanford that we often spent hours going from department
to department visiting the doctors, nurses and other caregivers.
Stanford had practically been our home for a year-and-a-half.

5/17/93
Appt. @ LPCH@S. Clinic D
Blood work
Urine to Oklahoma—Yippee I.O.
Skin test in allergy clinic to check Kyle's immune system
Height- 89.5cm(35 1/4")
Weight- 13.8kg(31 1b)

CATS ARE NORMAL! ! !

HVA—16(0-22)

We graduate to 6 months between appointments!

Crossing another hurdle was very reassuring. We knew the further away from cancer, the better off we were. There were still
many more hurdles to go, but we were operating as a normal family with neuroblastoma living at the backs of our minds instead of
in the forefronts. We were able to concentrate on living and enjoying everyday life.

With our lives on an even keel, I told Richmond I would like to visit Kendra before she died. I would have to take Haley since she was still nursing, but that was OK. Babies made everybody smile, anyway. (At least babies who aren't screaming.)

When Kendra and I spoke on the phone, I told her I'd like to come out for a visit to Fort Collins. A long weekend would be nice. The timing was important, so I inquired when would be best.

"You could come in two weeks," Kendra replied, "but four weeks from now...might not be a good time."

Her mom, Sharon, was in Fort Collins helping take care of Kendra. Her dad, David, and sister were also there, although not on the weekend I visited. She wanted to die at home, so they brought all the necessary hospital paraphernalia to make it work. Her boyfriend, Tom, was also there. He and Kendra had been sweethearts since she was about 15. He stuck by her side the whole time. He was a wonderful young man at only 18 years of age.

Richmond hugged Haley and me as we left for the airport. He knew that Kendra had given us all incredible inspiration and hope. It was my turn to be there for her. I was afraid that many of her friends might not have the courage to visit her. I was afraid myself, but knew, regardless, I would be glad to see her. A body riddled with cancer is a frightening sight. She and her family were living with that every day. I had to go tell her in person how important she had been to me and that I loved her. I had to thank her for being a part of our lives.

6/3/94 and 6/4/94
We (Haley and I) are here in Fort Collins. This is a very good, but very hard visit. It is so painful seeing Kendra in pain and covered with tumors. She can only move half of her body now, but is keeping her same spirit saying, "I'm not a vegetable, I'm only 1/2 a vegetable."

She is incredible. We are overwhelmed with sadness for her and her family. She said, "I'm not afraid of death...I'm just curious."

The weekend Kendra and I spent visiting together was one I will never forget. Her body was shutting down, but her spirit soared. After finding out she had a great respect for Native American culture, I told her about a dream that Richmond had a few months before. He dreamed that Kendra was talking to a medicine man and she had her hair ball. A moment later she was gone and an eagle soared up in the sky. It was a very peaceful dream, and after I told Kendra the story she said, "That makes me feel so peaceful inside."

Sharon and I talked together a lot that weekend. I asked Sharon if she had anything that she thought could help other parents in a similar situation. She reflected, then said:

"You always have to give it your best shot, and try to look for the good (in your child). They need to hear it and you need to say it."

The biggest lesson, "There are no guarantees," was followed by another thought from Sharon: "Love each other and show your love for your child. Take it one day at a time."

Sharon and David were wonderful parents. They radiated courage and strength and passed it onto Kendra. I knew when I left I would never see her again.

She died June 19.

I NEEDED TO FOCUS on our blessings. Our family was intact with Anna, Kyle and Haley all growing bigger every day. Many of our friends from the hospital weren't as lucky. I still felt as though we had an ax hanging over our heads and always hoped the cord would not be cut.

Our appointment that followed also left us with new fears. An echocardiogram was done to check for damage that can manifest itself as the heart muscle grows, as a result of using Adriamycin (chemo). Kyle also had some freckles examined by the dermatologist to check for skin cancer in the radiated area.

Kyle's immune system was recovering, although his nose ran every day. The immunologist did a series of blood tests, finding the only immune area that was low affected his ear, nose and throat. For that there was a vaccine.

Kyle had no treatments for almost three years. The journal entries were as follows.

5/1/94

The last 10 days have been boogers. I am always an optimist, but am now afraid to be. I hate the waiting and not knowing. I know too much and too many that have died to not be afraid. I don't want to live at the hospital, and I don't want to be away from RHB, Anna and Haley. Please dear God, let Kyle be clear and give us strength.

5/12/94

I hate waiting for cat (catecholamine) results. I hate it!

5/17/94

Kyle's tests are NORMAL! ! We have dodged another bullet. No one has cut the string holding the hatchet. Thank God!

Having the journal was like having a friend to talk to no matter what time it was or what I wanted to talk about. Talking about cancer scares the hell out of some people—and rightfully so. It's a mystefying and unforgiving disease.

To this date, Kyle's continued good health blesses our lives with family togetherness and great hopes for the future.

Where Do We Go From Here?

It's been eight years since Kyle has had any treatments. And eight years in remission—which leaves us functioning as normal as any family.

Most days, fear is nestled in the backs of our minds. We give barely a conscious thought to cancer as we continue on with work, and all the other pieces of a family's day. The disease crosses my mind every morning as I give Kyle his hearing aids to put in, knowing they are required due to the cisplatin chemotherapy. Otherwise, I direct the same thoughts toward my son as most other moms: don't pick your nose; pick up your shoes; don't pick on your sisters.

As checkups come and go, I can see that the fear will never be gone.

As I write this, we are waiting for periodic results, and the tension in my neck is present. I find myself screaming at the kids for being themselves, and I know in my heart what I really want is to wring cancer's neck with my bare hands so it can never, ever grow again. Each time Kyle goes for an annual checkup (which will be ongoing for the rest of his life), Richmond and I find our own ways of dealing with the possibility that he could be back in the throes of cancer. I have found myself engulfed in raging fear as I pray that we won't have to go back and live in the cancer ward.

Richmond generally decides it really isn't bothering him for about two weeks, at which point he says, "You know…maybe that's why I've been so edgy lately." It takes us awhile to come to terms with the idea of it even being possible again, and that brings us face to face with all the old bogeymen.

As far as the kids are concerned, the hospital is a great place to visit. Although Anna had a few horrific dreams, she claims she really doesn't think about it much. She enjoys all the nurses at Stanford as they've watched her grow up. Kyle absolutely loves the hospital and each hug and kiss he gets. Haley is simply happy to go along for the ride.

On days when I start getting upset about something insignificant, I often pause and contemplate how much more difficult life could be. And how incredibly happy I am that it's not.

DONNA L. BREEN SEPT. 9, 1999

GLOSSARY

ANC (Absolute Neutrophil Count): A count of the most common type of granulocytic white blood cell, neutrophils are responsible for much of the body's protection against infection. An inadequate number of neutrophils (neutropenia) leaves the body at high risk for infection from many sources.

Adriamycin: An antineoplastic drug used in chemotherapy.

anesthesia: Administration of an anesthetic agent to achieve partial or complete loss of sensation, with or without loss of consciousness.

bactrim: An antibiotic.

bands: An early-stage white blood cell count when determining an absolute neutrophil count.

bone biopsy: Excision of a small piece bone for microscopic examination using a hollow needle.

bone marrow: The soft organic material that fills the cavities of the bone.

bone marrow biopsy: Excision of a small piece of bone marrow for microscopic examination by use of a syringe and needle.

bone scan: The use of short half-life radiopharmaceutical agents to visualize bones. Especially useful in delineating osteomyelitis and metastases to the bone.

CAT scan: An image made with computerized tomography

CH@S: Childrens Hospital at Stanford, Palo Alto, Calif. (Closed June 1991 to make way for LPCH@S.)

chloral hydrate: Most commonly used to induce sleep.

Cisplatin: An antineoplastic chemical used in treating testicular tumors and ovarian cancer—a chemotherapy.

Cytoxan: Trade name for cyclophosphamide (a chemotherapy).

cyclophosphamide: An effective antineoplastic agent that has also been used as an immunosuppressive agent in organ transplantation. Trade name: Cytoxan.

echocardiogram: The graphic record produced by echocardiography (a non-invasive diagnostic method that uses ultrasound to visualize internal cardiac structures).

F&N: (Fever and Neutropenia): When a patient's fever is elevated and accompanied by an abnormally small number of neutrophil (infection-fighting) cells in the blood.

ganglionueroma: A neuroma containing ganglion cells. (A mature neuroblastoma that isn't malignant.)

Glycopyrroat: Useful with general anesthetics to dry secretions.

halothane: A fluorinated hydrocarbon used as a general anesthetic.

hemoglobin: The iron-containing pigment of the red blood cells. Its function is to carry oxygen from the lungs to the tissues.

heparin (heparin lock flush solution): A standard solution of heparin sodium, USP, labeled to indicate it is intended for maintenance of patency of intravenous injection devices only.

Hickman: A permanent IV access. The tube runs from the center of the chest, under the skin toward the neck where it goes down a large main vein into the heart. It is used to administer medications, draw blood or give transfusions, eliminating painful blood draws or shots.

IV: intravenous(ly) In the veins.

catecholamines: A urine test that measures vanillic acids (an indicator for neuroblastoma).

ketamine (ketamine hydrochloride): A non-barbiturate substance that is used intravenously or intramuscularly to produce anesthesia. The patient becomes cataleptic and may appear to be awake, but is unaware of the environment and unresponsive to pain.

LPCH@S: Lucile Salter Packard Children's Hospital at Stanford, Palo Alto, Calif. (opened June 1991).

monos (monocytes): They make up 3 to 8 percent of all white blood cells.

MRI (Magnetic Resonance Imaging): When certain atomic nuclei with an odd number of protons or neutrons or both are subjected to a strong magnetic field, they absorb and re-emit electromagnetic energy.Analysis of the net magnetization vector's deflection by application of a radiofrequency pulse provides image information.This technique (bouncing magnetic energy off the body) is valuable in providing images of the heart, large blood vessels, brain and soft tissues.

NPO: non per os (Latin), nothing by mouth. (Nothing to eat or drink)

ET tube (endotracheal tube): When laryngeal reflexes are depressed, tube is used inside the trachea to provide an airway (allowing the patient to breathe) while preventing aspiration of foreign material in the bronchus.

neuroblastoma: A malignant tumor composed principally of cells resembling neuroblasts that give rise to cells of the sympathetic system, especially adrenal medulla. Occurs chiefly in infants and children. Primary sites are in the mediastinum (cavity between two principal portions of an organ) and retroperitoneum (the membrane lining the abdominal cavity) regions.

neutrophils: 60 percent of all white blood cells (WBCs) are neutorphils and play the most active role in fighting infection. These are the cells used in the ANC calculation.

platelets: A round disk found in the blood. Platelets play an important role in blood coagulation. When a small vessel is injured, platelets adhere to each other and the edges of the injury and form a plug that covers the area.The plug of blood clot soon retracts and stops the loss of blood.

polys: Polymorphonuclear (a multi-lobed white blood cell). One type of blood cell counted when determining an absolute neutrophil count.

propofol: A general anesthetic.

POG: Pediatric Oncology Group

rhabdomyosarcoma: A malignant neoplasm originating in skeletal muscle.

radiation: Ionizing radiation used for diagnostic or therapeutic purposes.

rads: Radiation absorbed doses.

segs: (same as polys).

spiked: When the patient's fever rises, he or she has spiked a fever.

T-Cell leukemia: An acute disease of unregulated clonal proliferation of the cells of the blood forming tissues. A blood disease.

transfusion: The injection of blood or a blood component into the bloodstream.

VP16: A chemotherapy.

Versed: Trade name for midazolam hydrochloride.(A benzodiazepine used to produce sedation for brief diagnostic or endoscopic procedures and as sedation prior to general anesthesia.) A drug that makes the patient sleepy and wipes out memory.

WBC: White blood count; white blood cells.

XRT (X-Ray therapy): Radiation therapy

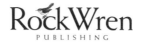

RockWren
PUBLISHING

O R D E R F O R M

Please send ___ copies of *Cancer's Gift* to:

_____
Company Name

_____
Name

_____
Address

_____
City   State   Zip

(____)____-_____   _____
Telephone   e-mail

Shipping
Book Rate: $2.00 for the first book and $1.00 for each additional book. (Surface shipping may take three to four weeks.)
Priority Mail: $4.75 for the first book and $2.00 for each additional book.

Payment
$12.95 per copy + shipping and handling. Please add 7.25% sales tax for books shipped to Nevada addresses. I understand that I may return any books for a full refund.

◯ Check Enclosed   ◯ VISA   ◯ MasterCard

_____   ____/____
Card Number   Exp. Date

_____
Name on Card

Fax Orders
775-829-4459

Telephone Orders
Toll free: 1-877-481-8248
Have your VISA or MasterCard ready

Postal Orders
Rock Wren Publishing
P.O. Box 70326, Reno, NV 89570-0326

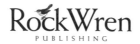

ROCK WREN

PUBLISHING

O R D E R   F O R M

Please send _____ copies of *Cancer's Gift* to:

_____
Company Name

_____
Name

_____
Address

_____
City   State   Zip

(_____)_____-_____   _____
Telephone   e-mail

Shipping
Book Rate: $2.00 for the first book and $1.00 for each additional book. (Surface shipping may take three to four weeks.)
Priority Mail: $4.75 for the first book and $2.00 for each additional book.

Payment
$12.95 per copy + shipping and handling. Please add 7.25% sales tax for books shipped to Nevada addresses. I understand that I may return any books for a full refund.

○ Check Enclosed   ○ VISA   ○ MasterCard

_____   _____/_____
Card Number   Exp. Date

_____
Name on Card

Fax Orders
775-829-4459

Telephone Orders
Toll free: 1-877-481-8248
Have your VISA or MasterCard ready

Postal Orders
Rock Wren Publishing
P.O. Box 70326, Reno, NV 89570-0326